60

Veterinary Technician's Handbook of Laboratory Procedures

Withdrawn

Veterinary Technician's Handbook of Laboratory Procedures

Brianne Bellwood

Melissa Andrasik-Catton

636.089607 BELLWOO 2014

Bellwood, Brianne,

Veterinary technician's
handbook of laboratory

WILEY Blackwell

Library Resource Center
Renton Technical College
3000 N.E. 4th Street
Renton, WA 98056

This edition first published 2014 © 2014 by John Wiley & Sons, Inc.

Editorial offices: 1606 Golden Aspen Drive, Suites 103 and 104, Ames, Iowa 50014-8300, USA
The Atrium, Southern Gate, Chichester, West Sussex, PO19 8SQ, UK
9600 Garsington Road, Oxford, OX4 2DQ, UK

For details of our global editorial offices, for customer services and for information about how to apply for permission to reuse the copyright material in this book please see our website at www.wiley.com/wiley-blackwell.

Authorization to photocopy items for internal or personal use, or the internal or personal use of specific clients, is granted by Blackwell Publishing, provided that the base fee is paid directly to the Copyright Clearance Center, 222 Rosewood Drive, Danvers, MA 01923. For those organizations that have been granted a photocopy license by CCC, a separate system of payments has been arranged. The fee codes for users of the Transactional Reporting Service are ISBN-13: 978-1-1183-4193-3/2014.

Designations used by companies to distinguish their products are often claimed as trademarks. All brand names and product names used in this book are trade names, service marks, trademarks or registered trademarks of their respective owners. The publisher is not associated with any product or vendor mentioned in this book.

The contents of this work are intended to further general scientific research, understanding, and discussion only and are not intended and should not be relied upon as recommending or promoting a specific method, diagnosis, or treatment by health science practitioners for any particular patient. The publisher and the author make no representations or warranties with respect to the accuracy or completeness of the contents of this work and specifically disclaim all warranties, including without limitation any implied warranties of fitness for a particular purpose. In view of ongoing research, equipment modifications, changes in governmental regulations, and the constant flow of information relating to the use of medicines, equipment, and devices, the reader is urged to review and evaluate the information provided in the package insert or instructions for each medicine, equipment, or device for, among other things, any changes in the instructions or indication of usage and for added warnings and precautions. Readers should consult with a specialist where appropriate. The fact that an organization or Website is referred to in this work as a citation and/or a potential source of further information does not mean that the author or the publisher endorses the information the organization or Website may provide or recommendations it may make. Further, readers should be aware that Internet Websites listed in this work may have changed or disappeared between when this work was written and when it is read. No warranty may be created or extended by any promotional statements for this work. Neither the publisher nor the author shall be liable for any damages arising herefrom.

Library of Congress Cataloging-in-Publication Data

Bellwood, Brianne, author.
   Veterinary technician's handbook of laboratory procedures / Brianne Bellwood, Melissa Andrasik-Catton.
      pages ; cm.
   Includes bibliographical references and index.
   ISBN 978-1-118-34193-3 (pbk. : alk. paper) – ISBN 978-1-118-72604-4 (epub) –
ISBN 978-1-118-72609-9 (emobi) – ISBN 978-1-118-72612-9 (epdf) – ISBN 978-1-118-73922-8 –
ISBN 978-1-118-73937-2   1. Veterinary clinical pathology–Laboratory manuals.
2. Veterinary medicine–Laboratory manuals.   I. Andrasik-Catton, Melissa, author.   II. Title.
   [DNLM: 1. Clinical Laboratory Techniques–veterinary–Handbooks.   2. Animal
Technicians–Handbooks.   SF 772.6]
   SF772.6.B45 2014
   636.089'607–dc23
                     2013024790

A catalogue record for this book is available from the British Library.

Wiley also publishes its books in a variety of electronic formats. Some content that appears in print may not be available in electronic books.

Cover design by Jen Miller Designs

Set in 9/12.5 pt Interstate Light by Toppan Best-set Premedia Limited

Printed and bound in Singapore by Markono Print Media Pte Ltd

1 2014

To my family, for the continued support and encouragement they've shown me in all my endeavors. To my past instructors, who instilled in me the passion for veterinary medicine and inspired me to pursue a teaching career. To my colleagues and students at Lakeland College, with whom I have had the privilege of sharing this passion.

Brianne Bellwood

I wish to thank my family for the unconditional support they've given me in living every aspect of my true passion. My training at Maple Woods Veterinary Technology School and the amazing veterinary community I have been privileged to grow with has provided me invaluable teachings; allowing me to share that knowledge with other technicians over these many exciting years.

Melissa Andrasik-Catton

Contents

Preface

Laboratory procedures are an essential diagnostic component of veterinary medicine. The role of the veterinary technician is to collect and process samples and then analyze and report the findings. This book provides a useful tool for reference when conducting many common laboratory tests, and serves as an excellent companion to full textbooks. The following chapters incorporate discussions on the use of common laboratory equipment, proper quality control methods, blood analysis, urinalysis, parasitology, and cytology.

Useful characteristics of this handbook, whether used in school or a clinic setting, are step-by-step procedures, discussions of common mistakes and errors, tips and tricks, and plenty of reference images. Color images are invaluable when trying to identify an unknown structure, and these are concisely provided in each chapter of this book.

In contrast to other texts available, this book provides needed information quickly and at a glance.

An accompanying website provides additional images and study tools for students, such as PowerPoint slides and crossword puzzles.

Brianne Bellwood
Melissa Andrasik-Catton

Acknowledgments

I would like to thank Lakeland College's Animal Health Technology Program and its staff and faculty for assistance in providing resources and samples for this book.

B.B.

I would like to thank Maple Woods Veterinary Technology Program for providing certain resources found in this book.

M.A.-C.

About the Companion Website

This book is accompanied by a companion website:
www.wiley.com/go/bellwoodhandbook

The website includes:

- Case studies provided in Powerpoint files
- Powerpoints of all figures from the book for downloading
- Crossword puzzles and answers as PDFs
- Video of an ear mite
- Powerpoints of additional figures for downloading

Veterinary Technician's Handbook of Laboratory Procedures

Chapter 1
Laboratory Equipment

Laboratory equipment

The variety of sophisticated laboratory equipment in a veterinary practice will depend largely on the size and scope of the practice itself. There are several pieces of core equipment that are expected in every practice that performs in-house testing and analysis.

Microscope

Purpose

The microscope is the most important piece of equipment in the veterinary clinic laboratory. The microscope is used to review fecal, urine, blood, and cytology samples on a daily basis (see Figure 1.1). Understanding how the microscope functions, how it operates, and how to care for it will improve the reliability of your results and prolong the life of this valuable piece of equipment.

Parts and functions of a compound microscope (Figure 1.1)

(A) **Arm:** Used to carry the microscope.

(B) **Base:** Supports the microscope and houses the light source.

(C) **Oculars (or eyepieces):** The lens of the microscope you look through. The ocular also magnifies the image. The total magnification can be calculated by multiplying the objective power by the ocular power. Oculars come in different magnifications, but 10× magnification is common.

(D) **Diopter adjustment:** The purpose of the diopter adjustment is to correct the differences in vision an individual may have between their left and right eyes.

(E) **Interpupillary adjustment:** This allows the oculars to move closer or further away from one another to match the width of an individual's eyes. When looking through the microscope, one should see only a single field of view. When viewing a sample, always use both eyes. Using one eye can cause eye strain over a period of time.

(F) **Nosepiece:** The nosepiece holds the objective lenses. The objectives are mounted on a rotating turret so they can be moved into place as needed. Most nosepieces can hold up to five objectives.

(G) **Objective lenses:** The objective lens is the lens closest to the object being viewed, and its function is to magnify it. Objective lenses are available in many powers, but

Veterinary Technician's Handbook of Laboratory Procedures, First Edition. Brianne Bellwood and Melissa Andrasik-Catton.
© 2014 John Wiley & Sons, Inc. Published 2014 by John Wiley & Sons, Inc.

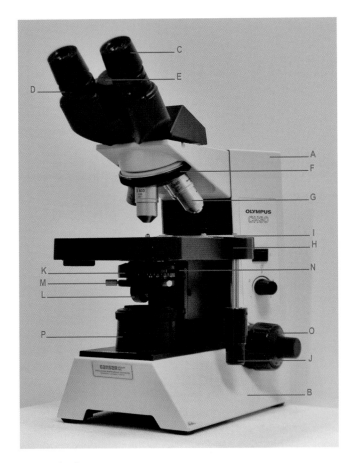

Figure 1.1 Compound microscope.

4×, 10×, 40×, and 100× are standard. 4× objective is used mainly for scanning. 10× objective is considered "low power," 40× is "high power" and 100× objective is referred to as "oil immersion."Once magnified by the objective lens, the image is viewed through the oculars, which magnify it further. Total magnification can be calculated by multiplying the objective power by the ocular lens power. For example:

100×objective lens with 10×oculars = 1000×total magnification.

(H) **Stage:** The platform on which the slide or object is placed for viewing.
(I) **Stage brackets:** Spring-loaded brackets, or clips, hold the slide or specimen in place on the stage.
(J) **Stage control knobs:** Located just below the stage are the stage control knobs. These knobs move the slide or specimen either horizontally (x-axis) or vertically (y-axis) when it is being viewed.

(K) **Condenser:** The condenser is located under the stage. As light travels from the illuminator, it passes through the condenser, where it is focused and directed at the specimen.

(L) **Condenser control knob:** Allows the condenser to be raised or lowered.

(M) **Condenser centering screws:** These crews center the condenser, and therefore the beam of light. Generally, they do not need much adjustment unless the microscope is moved or transported frequently.

(N) **Iris diaphragm:** This structure controls the amount of light that reaches the specimen. Opening and closing the iris diaphragm adjusts the diameter of the light beam.

(O) **Coarse and fine focus adjustment knobs:** These knobs bring the object into focus by raising and lowering the stage. Care should be taken when adjusting the stage height. When a higher power objective is in place (100× objective for example), there is a risk of raising the stage and slide and hitting the objective lens. This can break the slide and scratch the lens surface.

   Coarse adjustment is used for finding focus under low power and adjusting the stage height. Fine adjustment is used for more delicate, high power adjustment that would require fine tuning.

(P) **Illuminator:** The illuminator is the light source for the microscope, usually situated in the base. The brightness of the light from the illuminator can be adjusted to suit your preference and the object you are viewing.

Kohler illumination
What is Kohler illumination?
Kohler illumination is a method of adjusting a microscope in order to provide optimal illumination by focusing the light on the specimen. When a microscope is in Kohler, specimens will appear clearer, and in more detail.

Process of setting Kohler
Materials required
- Specimen slide (will need to focus under 10× power)
- Compound microscope.

Kohler illumination
(1) Mount the specimen slide on the stage and focus under 10×.
(2) Close the iris diaphragm completely.
(3) If the ball of light is not in the center, use the condenser centering screws to move it so that it is centered.
(4) Using the condenser adjustment knobs, raise or lower the condenser until the edges of the field becomes sharp (see Figure 1.2 and Figure 1.3).
(5) Open the iris diaphragm until the entire field is illuminated.

When should you set/check Kohler?
- During regular microscope maintenance
- After the microscope is moved/transported
- Whenever you suspect objects do not appear as sharp as they could be.

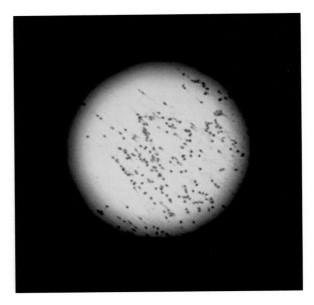

Figure 1.2   Note the blurry edges of the unfocused light.

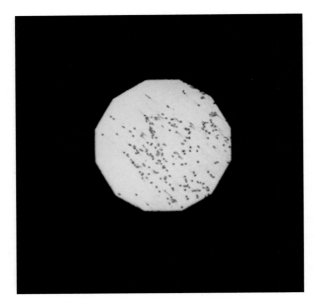

Figure 1.3   Adjusting the condenser height sharpens the edges of the "ball of light."

Microscope care and maintenance

Routine care and proper maintenance of microscope will ensure good performance over the years. In addition to this, a properly maintained and clean microscope will always be ready for use at any time. Professional cleaning and maintenance should be considered when routine techniques fail to produce optimal performance of the microscope.

Cleaning and maintenance supplies

Dust cover: When not in use, a microscope should be covered to protect it from dust, hair, and any other possible sources of dirt. It is important to note that a dust cover should never be placed over a microscope while the illuminator is still on.

Lens tissue: Lint-free lens tissues are delicate wipes that would not scratch the surface of the oculars or objective. Always ensure that you are using these types of tissues. Never substitute facial tissue or paper towel, as they are too abrasive.

Lens cleaner: Lens cleaning solution assists in removing fingerprints and smudges on lenses and objectives. Apply the lens cleaner to the lens tissue paper and clean/polish the surface.

Compressed air duster: Using compressed air to rid the microscope of dust particles is far superior to using your own breath and blowing onto the microscope. Compressed air is clean, and avoids possible contamination of saliva particles.

Maintenance tips

(1) Whenever the microscope is not in use, turn off the illuminator. This will greatly extend the life of the bulb, as well as keep the temperature down during extended periods of laboratory work.

(2) When cleaning the microscope, use distilled water or lens cleaner. Avoid using other chemicals or solvents, as they may be corrosive to the rubber or lens mounts.

(3) After using immersion oil, clean off any residue immediately. Avoid rotating the 40× objective through immersion oil. If this should occur, immediately clean the 40× objective with lens cleaner before the oil has a chance to dry.

(4) Do not be afraid to use many sheets of lens tissue when cleaning. Use a fresh piece (or a clean area of the same piece) when moving to a different part of the microscope. This avoids tracking dirt/oil/residue to other areas of the microscope.

(5) Store the microscope safely with the stage lowered and the smallest objective in position (4× or 10×). This placement allows for the greatest distance between the stage and the objective. If the microscope is bumped, the likelihood of an objective becoming damaged by the stage surface will be greatly minimized.

Troubleshooting

"I can focus my slide under 10×, but not under 40×."

A common reason for this is that the slide is upside down. Double check which side the smear is on (may not be the same side as the label!) and try focusing again.

Another cause could be dried immersion oil on the 40× objective that is obstructing your view. When switching from oil immersion (100×) to 40×, there is a good chance that the tip of the 40× objective could be dragged through some immersion oil. If it is not immediately cleaned off, it will dry, producing a thick haze.

To fix: Use lens paper and lens cleaner to clean the end of the 40× objective. This may need to be repeated several times depending on how thick the dried oil is. After cleaning, use a dry piece of lens paper to polish the objective.

To avoid the problem: Clean up oil immediately after use. Clean the end of the 100× objective and any heavy oil present on the slide before moving back down to 40× objective.

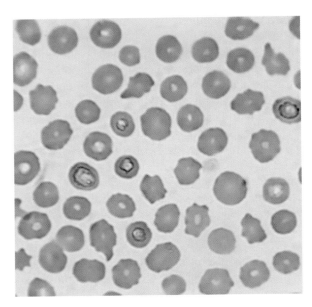

Figure 1.4 Water artifact seen on the surface of the red blood cells (1000× magnification).

"In hematology, when I focus under 40×, my red blood cells appear shiny."

This is most likely due to water artifact during the staining and drying process (see Figure 1.4). To make visualization of the cells easier, add a small drop of immersion oil to your slide. *Gently* spread the drop of oil over the area you will be examining. Wipe of excess oil using the side of your finger. *Be very gentle when doing this, and use a clean finger each time you wipe. Wiping too hard or rough will cause your smear to rub off.* This technique will leave a very thin layer of oil on your smear. The film is thin enough that you can use the 40× objective without running the risk of the lens becoming contaminated with oil.

Try focusing under 40× again, and the shininess should have been resolved.

"There's no light coming from the illuminator."

The first assumption is always that the bulb is burnt out, but it is a good idea to check a couple of other possibilities as well.

If the iris diaphragm is closed and the brightness of the illuminator is at its lowest, the light may be so small that it appears as if there is no light present.

Check to make sure the cord is fully plugged into the back of the microscope. This plug can become dislodged slightly during transport and microscope set up.

If your microscope is the type that uses fuses, it may be the fuse—not the bulb—that needs replacing.

When the microscope is not in use, be sure to turn it off. This will help prolong the life of the bulb.

Clean up

When the use of the microscope is complete, following proper clean up procedures will improve the quality of images that are viewed and extend the life of the microscope and its components:

(1) Remove the slide from the stage and dispose of it properly.
(2) Clean any oil residue or sample material that may have contaminated the stage surface.
(3) Lower the stage and move the smallest objective into place.
(4) Clean the objective lens and oculars after every use. The order in which they are cleaned is important. Cleaning the 100× objective first and then moving onto other parts will result in immersion oil being spread onto all other components. Using lens tissue and lens cleaner, begin with cleaning the oculars, then the 4× objective, the 10× objective, 40× objective, and finish with the 100× objective lens.

Centrifuge

Another key component of the veterinary laboratory is the centrifuge. Numerous centrifuge types exist for different purposes, such as those for microhematocrit, fecal, urine, and blood samples. It is not uncommon to use a multiuse centrifuge that can be set to spin at a speed appropriate for the biological sample, with specialized holding devices for each type of sample. The manufacturer's guide should be used for operation, maintenance, and cleaning instructions.

Microhematocrit centrifuge

This centrifuge is used exclusively for spinning down microhematocrit tubes (see Figure 1.5). This process is used for determining a patient's PCV (packed cell volume) or can also provide a plasma sample for protein analysis.

Clinical centrifuge

Clinical centrifuges are available in two main types: a variable angle centrifuge or a fixed angle centrifuge.

The variable angle centrifuge (also called a horizontal centrifuge) has swinging buckets that hold the specimen tubes. As the centrifugation begins, these buckets swing out horizontally, and the particles within the specimen are pushed to the base of the tube to form the sediment (see Figure 1.6). Once the rotation stops, the buckets return to their upright position. This change of position from horizontal to vertical can result in a slight remixing of the sample. This effect should be taken into consideration when preparing a sample.

The fixed angle centrifuge has buckets that are in a fixed position, typically about 50° (see Figure 1.7). The specimen tubes are held in this position for the entire centrifugation process.

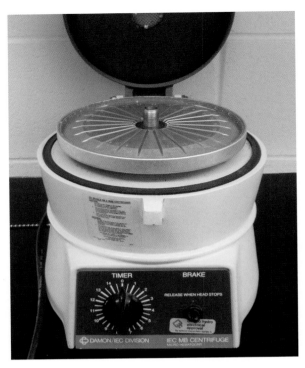

Figure 1.5   Microhematocrit centrifuge. This centrifuge is used for spinning microhematocrit tubes only. It is preset to 10,000 rpm.

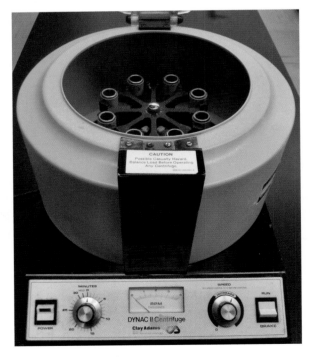

Figure 1.6   Variable angle centrifuge. Buckets swing out horizontally during the centrifugation process.

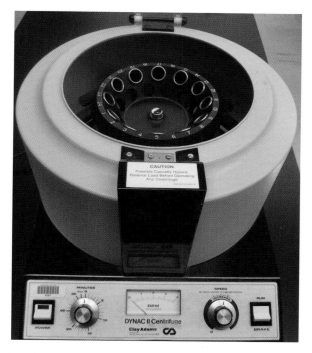

Figure 1.7 Fixed angle centrifuge. Buckets are at a fixed angle (typically about 50°) and do not move during the centrifugation process.

StatSpin

Another option is the StatSpin (see Figure 1.8). This centrifuge is a fixed angle centrifuge designed for small samples. It has a faster spinning speed, and as a result, a shorter processing time. These qualities could be beneficial in a small animal or exotic veterinary practice.

Refractometer

The purpose of a refractometer is to measure the refractive index of a solution. When measuring a solution (i.e., urine), light passes through the sample and bends. The angle of this refraction is visualized as a shadow and correlates to the concentration of the solution. Veterinary specific refractometers are now on the market allowing for minor differences between dog and cat urine specific gravity and total protein values (see Figure 1.9).

The most common use of a refractometer in veterinary laboratories is to measure urine specific gravity and plasma total protein. Refractometers have built-in scales to measure both of these, and some brands of refractometers will also possess a refractive index scale. This scale, with the use of an appropriate conversion chart, can be used to measure the concentration of many other solutions.

Tips: Cover the entire prism with the liquid (urine or plasma) being examined. Reading urine and plasma at room temperature will provide the most accurate results.

Library Resource Center
Renton Technical College
3000 N.E. 4th Street
Renton, WA 98056

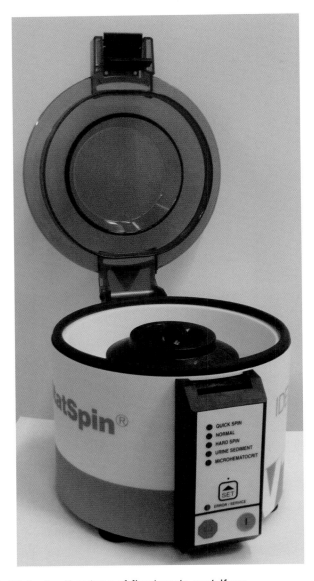

Figure 1.8 StatSpin. Another type of fixed angle centrifuge.

Calibration

It is good practice to calibrate the refractometer at the beginning of each day. This is achieved by applying a large drop of distilled water on the prism and adjusting the blue/white line to read exactly 1.000 on the scale. The adjustment knob or screw is located on various places of a refractometer; therefore, the manufacturer's guide will need to be consulted.

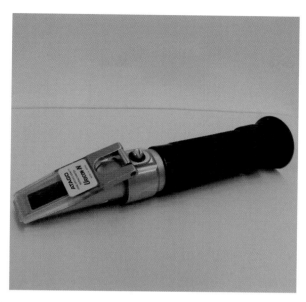

Figure 1.9   Refractometer.

Chemistry analyzers

There are a wide variety of chemistry analyzers available for veterinary use. Most use the principles of photometry to quantify analytes, such as enzymes, proteins, and other constituents in the blood. Electrochemical methods are used to analyze ionic compounds such as electrolytes. These two methods may require the use of two separate analyzers, or they may be combined into one.

Another variation among analyzers is the way they facilitate the photometry testing procedure. A sample needs to be added to a substrate to initialize the test. Examples include slides, rotors, or cartridges (see Figure 1.10).

Depending upon the analyzer or the analyte being tested, a serum or plasma sample is required. Some analyzers have the ability to process whole blood sample as well. The type of anticoagulant recommended should be confirmed by reviewing the manufacturer recommendations.

Regardless of the analyzer type chosen, it is important to maintain the equipment according to the manufacturer's recommendations. With such a wide variety of analyzers available, this book cannot describe the operation, maintenance, and cleaning of each brand. The manufacturer's guide should be consulted for this information. Regular maintenance is essential for ensuring the precision and accuracy of the analyzer. It may also be necessary for complying with the manufacturer's warranty.

Hematology analyzers

As with chemistry analyzers, there are many types of hematology analyzers to choose from. There are several different types of technology used to quantify cell types, and

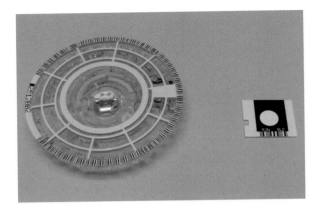

Figure 1.10 Testing supplies for various types of chemistry analyzers.

each has its own advantages and disadvantages. Examples of the technologies used are impedance, laser-based, and optical fluorescence. An analyzer may use one, or a combination of these technologies to detect and enumerate the cells present in the sample.

While the analyzers can provide a large amount of information about the patient, it is recommended to follow up with a manual examination to confirm readings, and review morphologies.

Coagulation analyzers

In-house coagulation testing is available to screen for coagulation disorders and measure fibrinogen levels. Tests such as prothrombin time (PT), activated partial thromboplastin time (aPTT), and fibrinogen can be performed using fresh or citrated whole blood.

As with all analyzers, it is recommended to follow appropriate maintenance and quality control procedures to ensure the accuracy and precision of the equipment.

Quality control of all laboratory equipment

Because diagnoses and treatment plans are made based on laboratory findings, it is imperative that the equipment utilized in the lab be in excellent working order, serviced at regular intervals, calibrated and cleaned as recommended by the manufacturer, and used properly. In addition to properly functioning equipment, there are things the technician can do to improve the accuracy of their test results:

(1) Follow manufacturer directions precisely.
(2) Become familiar with normal and abnormal findings.
(3) Log all activity of equipment, including daily, weekly, and monthly servicing.

(4) Standardize test methods within the hospital.
  (a) Perform urinalysis, fecal analysis, packed cell volume and total protein analysis, and cytology in the same manner no matter who is conducting the test.
(5) Save enough sample to perform tests more than once to verify accuracy of findings.

Remember, all laboratory equipment and its results are only as reliable as the human operating the equipment!

Chapter 2
Blood Analysis

Hematology

Proper blood collection and handling techniques

Blood is collected from animals in order to conduct many tests, ranging from hematology parameters to clinical chemistries, and even to evaluate coagulation disorders. Good technique when obtaining blood samples is important to maximize the reliability of the results.

Blood can be collected from many sites on animals; however, the most common for mammals is the jugular, cephalic, and lateral and medial saphenous veins. Reptilian, amphibian, and avian species have different locations for blood collection specific to the species. It is important to collect a sufficient quantity of blood for all the tests to be conducted.

Blood can be drawn utilizing a syringe and needle or a vacutainer system. The vacutainer technique is preferred, as this reduces the chance for a clotted sample, draws the accurate amount into the tube, and is considered sterile. Anticoagulant blood tubes should be gently inverted a number of times immediately after collection. Utilizing a blood rocking machine may be useful; however, overmixing or prolonged mixing of a sample can cause cellular damage.

Some tests require an anticoagulated sample (whole blood) or plasma, while others require serum. Whole blood samples are a representation of all the cells, liquid, and compounds within the blood mixed in a solution that will not allow the sample to clot. This can be spun down in a centrifuge to separate the cells (white blood cell [WBC], red blood cell [RBC], etc.) from the liquid (plasma); but remember, even when spun down, the sample has not clotted, it is just separated. Serum is often used for chemistries and is the liquid portion of a blood sample *after* it has clotted. The difference between plasma and serum is the clotting factors, primarily fibrinogen. Plasma has them, but serum does not, because those clotting factors are caught up in the clot.

Blood collection tubes

The tubes used to collect both types of samples (anticoagulated = whole blood and plasma; clotted = serum) come in many different colors and contents. It is important to

Veterinary Technician's Handbook of Laboratory Procedures, First Edition. Brianne Bellwood and Melissa Andrasik-Catton.
© 2014 John Wiley & Sons, Inc. Published 2014 by John Wiley & Sons, Inc.

maintain the proper blood:anticoagulant ratio when collecting a sample. Underfilling a blood tube can result in sample dilution by the anticoagulant itself. Here are common tubes used in veterinary medicine, the color of the tube, what is in it, and what it's used for:

Note: The following tubes come in many different colors depending on the source. It is not unusual to find human blood tubes with different colors. READ LABELS.

Purple top: Ethylenediaminetetraacetic acid (EDTA) anticoagulant—for a complete blood count (CBC) (not all machines), mammalian blood smear, plasma for specific tests, and blood typing.

Green top: Sodium or lithium heparin anticoagulant—for CBC (not all machines), avian/reptilian/amphibian blood smear, and plasma for specific tests.

Red top: Plain—for clotting a blood sample but does not separate the clot from the serum. Serum is used to run chemistries. Red tops are often used for sterile urine collection and other bodily fluids.

Gray and red top (tiger top, marble top): Plain with silicone gel separator—for clotting a blood sample; separates the clot from the serum. Used for most tests requiring serum. Some tests require no gel separator during centrifugation and transportation. Use a plain red top in these cases.

Blue top: Sodium citrate—for coagulation profiles on any species.

Gray top: Diatomaceous earth or kaolin—for activated clotting times.

Gray top: Boric acid—urine preservative. Preserves cellular material in urine, but you must run a dip-stick prior to placing urine in this tube.

Tips

When performing hematology tests on mammalian samples, blood should be collected in EDTA anticoagulant blood tubes. Heparin anticoagulant is preferred when performing hematology evaluations on avian or reptilian/amphibian blood, but Heparin anticoagulant can have its uses in mammalian hematology as well. An extracellular RBC parasite, *Mycoplasma*, has the tendency to fall off the cells when exposed to EDTA. Using heparinized blood can make the identification of Mycoplasma easier. If hemoparasites are suspected, identification can be made easier by using fresh blood for the smear, immediately after collection, before any anticoagulant is added. Using fresh blood immediately after collection will also decrease platelet clumping.

Peripheral blood smears

Purpose

Preparing a peripheral blood smear (PBS) allows for microscopic examination of blood cells. On a well-made PBS, cells can be easily counted and their morphological characteristics evaluated accurately.

The goal of a PBS is to obtain a "monolayer." The monolayer is an area of the smear where cells are evenly distributed, not spread too far apart or overlapping. The majority of counts and evaluations will be performed in this area, also known as the "read area."

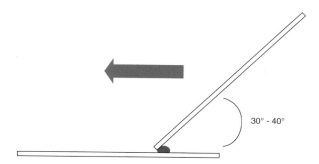

30° - 40°

Figure 2.1   Technique for preparing a peripheral blood smear.

Materials required
- Well-mixed anticoagulated whole blood
- Glass microscope slides
- Capillary tube
- Lens tissue.

Procedure
(1) It is important to begin with two clean, dust free microscope slides. If slides are dirty or dusty, polish them using lint-free lens tissue.
(2) Using a capillary tube, obtain a sample of whole blood. Ensure that the blood is well mixed by gently inverting it several times before sampling with the capillary tube.
(3) If blood is not well mixed, cells begin to settle causing the cell distribution on your PBS to be inaccurate.
(4) Place a small drop of blood (2-3 mm) at the end of your slide.
(5) The second slide is used as a "spreader" slide and should be held at a 30°-40° angle. See "Tips" below for additional points.
(6) Using a thumb and forefinger, anchor the bottom slide to the counter and back the spreader slide into the blood drop. (see Figure 2.1)
(7) Pause at the blood drop for a brief second, and in a smooth fluid motion, advance the spreader slide to the end.
(8) Be sure not to change your angle or lift the spreader slide off of the bottom slide.

There are many techniques for creating a smear. Different methods should be practiced to determine which is most comfortable for the technician.

Characteristics of a good smear (See Figure 2.2)
- Covers 3/4 of the slide
- Symmetrical, bullet-shape
- No tails or ridges
- Microscopically: should have an even distribution of cells.

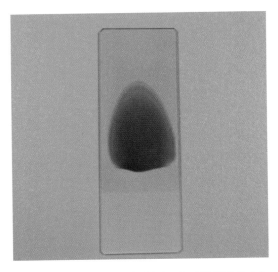

Figure 2.2 Example of a good quality PBS. Stained with Diff-Quick.

Troubleshooting

Table 2.1 Common errors in preparing a blood smear.

Error	Description	Cause/tips
Figure 2.3 "Tails" present on feathered edge.	Tails	Tails may be caused by lifting the spreader slide up at the end of the spreading motion. Debris present on the slide. Tails can also be the result of nicks in the edge of the spreader slide.

Table 2.1 *(Continued)*

Error	Description	Cause/tips
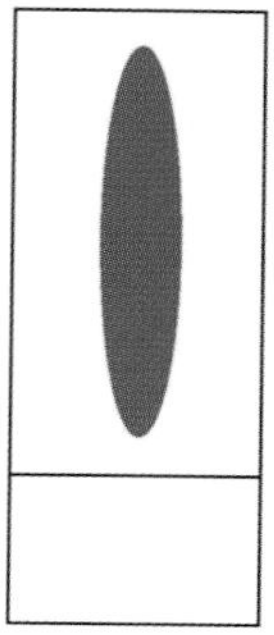	Long and narrow	Results when pushing the blood drop too soon before the blood has spread along the edge of the spreader slide. To fix: • Pause longer when backing into the drop. • Slow your speed slightly when moving the spreader slide forward.
Figure 2.4 Long and narrow.		
	Short and wide	If the spreader slide is held at an angle greater than 30°, the blood is not pushed out over the length of the slide. This causes a small, narrow monolayer. • Spreading too fast
Figure 2.5 Short and wide.		
	Square	When backing into the drop, the pause was too long Forward spreading speed was too slow
Figure 2.6 Square.		

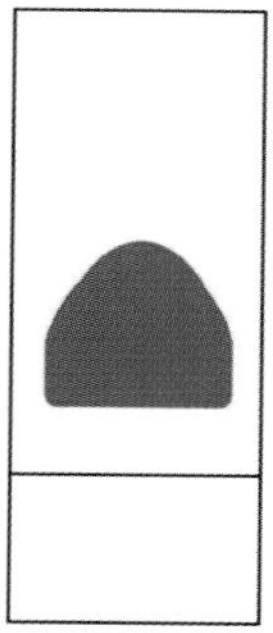

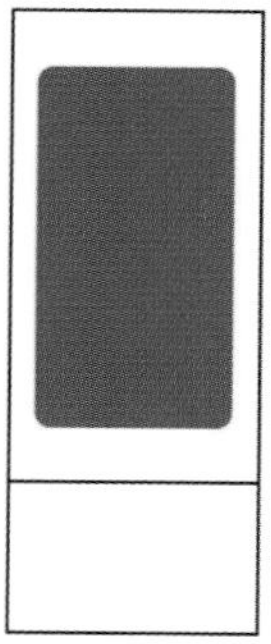

(Continued)

Table 2.1 (*Continued*)

Error	Description	Cause/tips
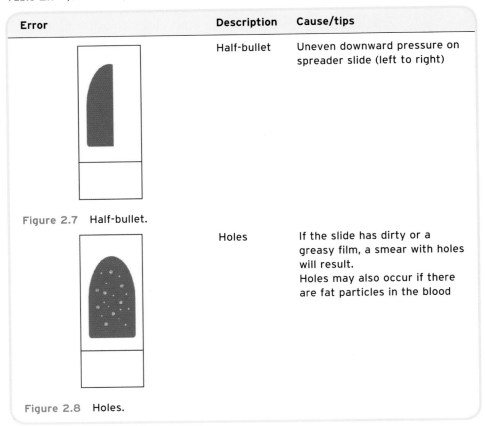	Half-bullet	Uneven downward pressure on spreader slide (left to right)

Figure 2.7 Half-bullet.

Holes	If the slide has dirty or a greasy film, a smear with holes will result. Holes may also occur if there are fat particles in the blood

Figure 2.8 Holes.

Tips

The blood of an anemic or dehydrated patient may be thinner or thicker than usual. Adjusting to a higher angle will help make a better smear from an anemic patient where lowering the angle when using thicker blood will help spread out the cells.

Staining

After a smear has completely air dried, it must be stained to identify cells and their characteristics. A Romanowsky-type stain, Wright's stain, is used in hematology to stain blood smears. A commercial stain that is commonly used is Diff-Quick, which is a modified Wright's stain (see Figure 2.9).

The stain consists of three solutions that fix and stain various components of the cells. The first solution, a fixative, consists of 95% methanol. The second solution, eosin, has an acidic pH and stains cell cytoplasms and eosinophilic granules. The third solution, methylene blue, has an alkaline pH and stains the nuclei of the cells.

The slide exposure time to each solution varies slightly depending upon the desired result or sample being stained. Typically, dipping a slide into each solution five times

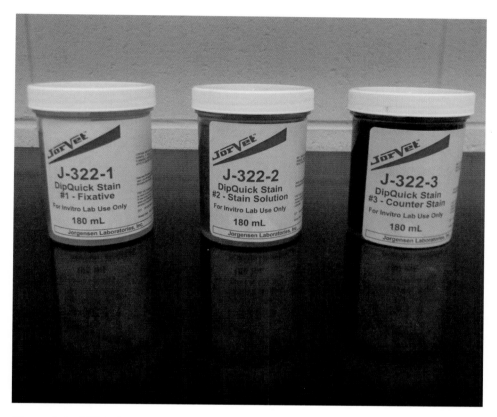

Figure 2.9 Diff-Quick stain set (DipQuick).

for one second each time dip will give adequate staining. This can be adjusted to alter the appearance of cells. It is important to rinse the slide after the last dip into stain #3. Distilled water is preferred. The now stained smear should be allowed to air dry. Rapid drying, such as a hair dryer or waving the slide, will cause crenation (distortion) of the RBCs.

Tip: Have one set of stains for blood and "clean" cytology specimens. Keep another set of "dirty" stains for fecal and ear cytology.

Tip: Old stain may precipitate, causing artifacts to appear on your smear. Replace/ Filter stain routinely depending upon usage.

Packed cell volume (PCV)

Materials required
- Well-mixed, anticoagulated whole blood
- Clay
- Reader card
- Centrifuge
- Capillary tubes.

Procedure

(1) Begin with well-mixed, anticoagulated blood.

(2) Fill two capillary tubes 3/4 full with blood, and seal one end with clay. Filling a second tube serves two purposes:

    (a) Serves as a counterbalance for centrifugation

    (b) Serves as a quality control to ensure accuracy.

(3) Place tubes in the groves of the centrifuge, directly across from one another, with the clay pointing towards the outside (see Figure 2.10).

(4) Close centrifuge lid(s).

Speed: 10,000 rpm

  Time: 5 minutes.

(Speed and time may vary depending on the unit.)

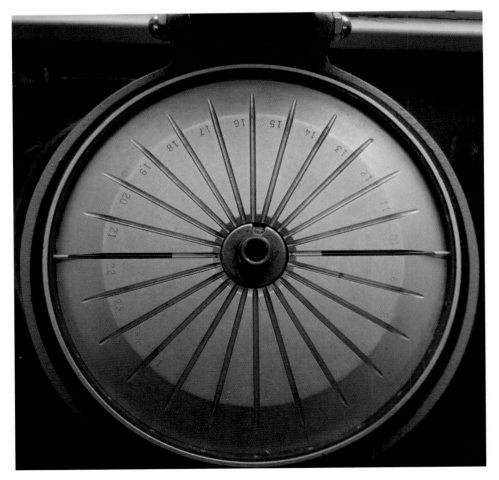

Figure 2.10 Proper placement of PCV tubes into a microhematocrit centrifuge.

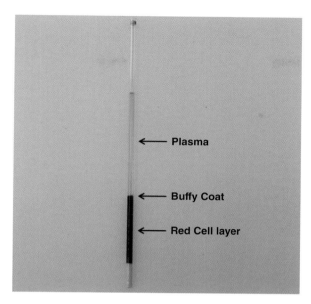

Figure 2.11 Layers of a PCV after centrifugation: plasma, buffy coat, and red cell layer.

Readings

After centrifugation, the blood in the microhematocrit tubes is separated into three layers: the plasma layer, the buffy coat layer, and the red cell layer (see Figure 2.11).

Using a reader card, align the top of the plasma layer with the 100 line, and the bottom of the red cell layer (between the red cells and the top of the clay) with the 0.

Measurement is taken at the top of the red cell layer where the red cells and plasma meet and is expressed as a percentage (see Figure 2.12).

Repeat for tube no. 2.

For quality control purposes, each reading should be within 1% of the average.

Sources of error

- Excessive anticoagulant in the blood sample.
- Using poorly mixed blood.
- Misalignment of tubes with the reader card.
- Including the buffy coat layer in your PCV measurement.
- Allowing the tubes to sit for more than 5 minutes prior to reading. The layers will begin to slant, making reading difficult.

Tip: **The hemoglobin value of a patient can be estimated by dividing the PCV reading by 3.**

Plasma evaluation

Total Protein (Total Serum Protein) can be assessed by utilizing the plasma portion of the PCV tube. One of the capillary tubes can be broken above the red cell line, and the

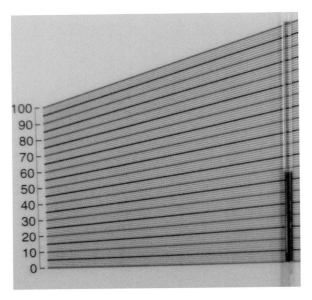

Figure 2.12   PCV reading technique. Note the bottom of the red cell layer is at 0 and the top of the plasma is at 100.

plasma (liquid) can be placed on a refractometer to determine the protein concentration. Depending on your type of refractometer, you will read the TP, SP or TS column and report the number in g/dL (g/100mL).

The color of plasma can yield information about the patient's health. Below are colors and associated disorders:

Normal: Clear or light straw-yellow (horses have very deep yellow)
Deep yellow plasma: Icteric; liver or hemolytic disorders
Red plasma: Hemolyzed; artificial from poor blood collection technique or hemolytic disorders
Milky plasma: Lipemic; artificial due to recent meal or high cholesterol and triglycerides, which may be due to liver or pancreatic issues.

A combination of these can be seen in samples from patients with multiple abnormalities.

Red blood cell count

Materials required
- Anticoagulated whole blood
- Ery-TIC test kit (Bioanalytic GmbH, Umkirch/Freiburg, Germany)
- Improved Neubauer hemocytometer (see Figure 2.13)
- Coverslip (specific for a hemocytometer)
- Microscope with 40× objective lens
- Cell counter.

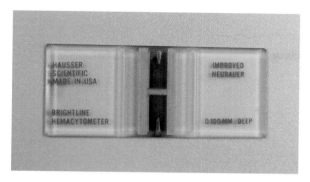

Figure 2.13   Improved Neubauer bemocytometer.

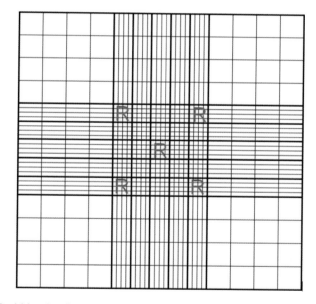

Figure 2.14   Red blood cell counting area, indicated by "R."

Procedure

(1) Follow Ery-TIC instructions for proper filling of the vial.

(2) Place the clean, hemocytometer-specific coverslip on top of the hemocytometer.

(3) Mix the Ery-TIC vial, and flood one side of the hemocytometer counting chamber using capillary action.

(4) Count the RBCs within five group squares (each consisting of 16 smallest squares) (see Figure 2.14).

(5) Repeat this count on the second side of the hemocytometer.

(6) Calculate totals for Side 1 and Side 2 of the hemocytometer grid.

Calculations and quality control

Calculations should be made using the average between Side 1 and Side 2.

QC: Side 1 and Side 2 totals should be within 10% of the average.

$$\frac{\text{Average} \times 10}{1000} = \underline{\quad} \times 10^6/\mu L$$

Sources of error

- Improper mixing of whole blood or prepared solution
- Improper filling of Ery-TIC vial
- Incomplete filling or overfilling of the hemocytometer chamber
- Using a dirty hemocytometer can cause difficulty with differentiating between RBCs and debris.

Red blood cell indices

Purpose

Calculating the RBC Indices can be a useful tool when examining cases of anemia. They can give insight to the size and hemoglobin concentration of the average RBC in the patient's sample. They are often used to determine the type of anemia. These are calculated when a CBC analyzer is used.

Information required

- Packed cell volume (L/L)
- Hemoglobin concentration (g/L)
- RBC count ($10^6/\mu L$).

MCV (mean corpuscular volume)

Being an indicator of volume, MCV can provide information regarding the size of the average RBC in a sample.

Formula:

$$\frac{\text{Packed Cell Volume (L/L)}}{\text{RBC Count } (10^6/\mu L)} \times 1000 = \underline{\quad} \text{fL}$$

Interpretation

Value lower than normal = microcytic: red cells are smaller than normal for that species.

Value higher than normal = macrocytic: red cells are larger than normal for that species.

MCH (mean corpuscular hemoglobin)

MCH can provide information regarding the weight of hemoglobin within the average RBC.

Formula:

$$\frac{\text{Hemoglobin (g/L)}}{\text{RBC Count } (10^6/\mu L)} = \underline{\quad} \text{pg}$$

Interpretation

Value lower than normal = red cells contain less than the average weight of hemoglobin for that species.

Value higher than normal = red cells contain more than the average weight of hemoglobin for that species.

MCHC (mean corpuscular hemoglobin concentration)

MCHC provides information regarding the concentration of hemoglobin within the average RBC. MCHC takes into account the amount of hemoglobin in proportion to the size of the average red cell.

Formula:

$$\frac{\text{Hemoglobin (g/L)}}{\text{Packed Cell Volume (L/L)}} = \underline{\quad} \text{g/L}$$

Interpretation

Value lower than normal = hypochromic: Average red cell contains a lower concentration of hemoglobin for that species

Value higher than normal = Average red cell contains a higher concentration of hemoglobin for that species.

Reticulocyte count

Purpose

Performing a reticulocyte count is indicated in cases of anemia, to determine whether the anemia is regenerative or not. A reticulocyte count should be performed on every anemic patient (except for horses, which do not release reticulocytes into circulation).

Important notes

Two forms of reticulocytes exist: punctate and aggregate (see Figure 2.15). In cats, only the aggregate forms should be counted.

Materials required

- New methylene blue (NMB) stain
- Whole blood
- Microscope slides
- Sterile red top tube
- Microscope with 100× objective
- Cell counter.

Procedure

Before preparing slides, the NMB stain should be filtered. This process will minimize artifacts such as stain precipitate, which may be falsely recorded as reticulocytes.

(1) Mix equal parts whole blood with filtered NMB stain in a sterile red top tube.
(2) Allow mixture to sit for 15–20 minutes, gently mixing every 5 minutes.
(3) Prepare two smears as you would for a PBS, and allow to air dry.

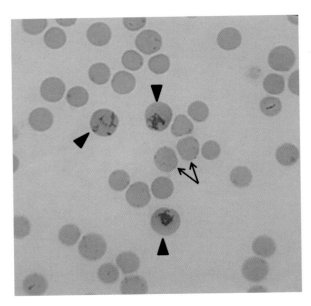

Figure 2.15   Punctate reticulocyte (arrow); aggregate reticulocyte (arrowhead).

(4) Reticulocyte counts are made by recording the number of reticulocytes seen per 500 RBCs under 1000× magnification.
(5) Repeat this process on smear no. 2.

Calculations and quality control
QC: Smear 1 and Smear 2 totals should be within 20% of each other before taking an average.

$$\text{Relative}: \frac{\text{Total(Slide 1+Slide 2)}}{1000} \times 100 = \underline{\quad} \%$$

$$\text{Absolute}: \frac{\text{Relative(\%)}}{100} \times \text{RBC Count } (10^6/\mu L) \times 1000 = \underline{\quad} \times 10^3/\mu L$$

Corrected reticulocyte percentage

Purpose
In cases of anemia, a reticulocyte percentage can be misleading, since the total number of RBCs is decreased. Correcting your reticulocyte percentage takes into account the decreased total mature RBC numbers circulating in the anemic patient.

Calculation

$$\text{Observed Retic } \% \times \frac{\text{Observed PCV}}{\text{Normal Species PCV}} = \underline{\quad} \%$$

For dogs: A PCV of 45% is used in the equation
For cats: A PCV of 35% is used in the equation.

Reticulocyte production index (RPI)

Purpose
Prematurely released reticulocytes have a longer life span than mature erythrocytes. Calculating the RPI accounts for this extended survival time and gives insight into whether the regenerative response to anemia is adequate.

Calculation:

$$RPI = \frac{\text{Corrected Retic \%}}{\text{Retic Maturation Time}}$$

Table 2.2   Reticulocyte maturation time factor.

Patient PCV	Maturation time factor
45%	1
35%	1.4
25%	2
15%	2.5

For example:

Corrected reticulocyte % = 5%
Patient's PCV = 15% (maturation time factor = 2.5).

$$RPI = \frac{5}{2.5} = 2$$

Table 2.3   Reticulocyte Production index (RPI) interpretation.

Dogs		
	RPI < 1	Nonregenerative anemia
	RPI 1-2	Responsive bone marrow
	RPI > 2	Accelerated erythropoiesis
	RPI ≥ 3	Significant regeneration

White blood cell count

Materials required
- Whole blood
- Leuko-TIC test kits (Bioanalytic GmbH)

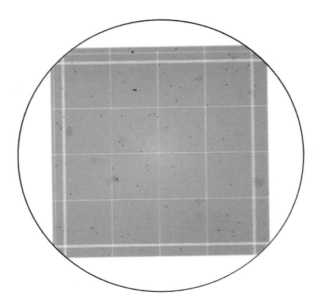

Figure 2.16 Microscopic view of hemocytometer grid with white blood cells.

- Improved Neubauer hemocytometer
- Coverslip (specifc for a hemocytometer)
- Microscope with 10× objective lens
- Cell counter.

Procedure

(1) Follow Leuko-TIC instructions for proper filling of the vial.
(2) Place a clean coverslip on top of the hemocytometer.
(3) Mix the Leuko-TIC vial, and flood one side of the hemocytometer counting chamber using capillary action.
(4) Using the 10× objective lens, count the WBCs contained within each the four big corner squares of the grid. (see Figure 2.16 and Figure 2.17).
(5) Repeat this count on the second side of the hemocytometer.
(6) Calculate totals for side 1 and side 2 of the hemocytometer grid.

Calculations and quality control

Calculations should be made using the average between Side 1 and Side 2.

QC: Side 1 and Side 2 totals should be within 10% of each other before taking the average.

$$\frac{\text{Average} \times 50}{1000} = \underline{\quad} 10^3/\mu L$$

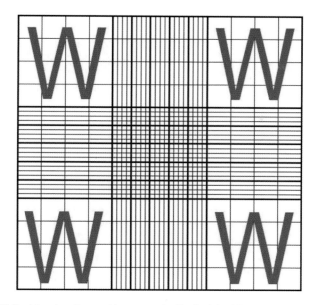

Figure 2.17   White blood cell counting area, indicated by "W."

Sources of error
- Improper mixing of whole blood or prepared solution
- Improper filling of Leuko-TIC vial
- Incomplete flooding over overfilling of the hemocytometer chamber
- Using a dirty hemocytometer can cause difficulty with differentiating between WBCs and debris.

White blood cell differential

Purpose
A WBC differential count gives us information regarding the proportion and numbers of individual leukocytes in the patient's sample, including significant morphological changes. This can provide useful diagnostic information in cases of inflammation, infection, and antigenic responses.

Materials required
- Stained PBS
- Microscope with 100× objective lens
- Cell counter.

Procedure
It is important that examination and counts be performed within the monolayer area of your slide (see Figure 2.18).

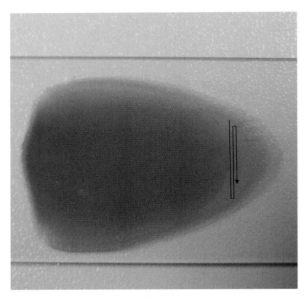

Figure 2.18   Read area (monolayer).

(1) Scan the slide in a methodical grid pattern, in order not to cover the same area twice.

   Counts can be completed quickly under 400× magnification, but if you are also evaluating morphology, 1000× magnification should be used.

(2) Count a minimum of 100 WBCs. *(If the total WBC Count is increased, 200 cells should be counted to maintain accuracy.)*

Calculations

Relative count:

$$\frac{\text{No. of Cell Type Seen}}{100} = \underline{\quad}\%$$

Absolute count:

$$\frac{\text{Relative (\%)}}{100} \times \text{WBC Count}\,(10^3/\mu L) = \underline{\quad} \times 10^3/\mu L$$

Note: Check your math:

- Relative counts of each cell type should add up to equal 100.
- Absolute counts of each cell type should add up to equal your WBC count.

White blood cell estimate

Purpose
Performing a WBC estimate can be useful as a quick evaluation of a patient's leukocyte numbers if the materials required for a count are not available. Estimates can also be done if an analyzer's WBC count is questionable or is flagged.

Materials required
- Stained PBS
- Microscope with 40× objective lens
- Cell counter.

Procedure
Examine a stained blood smear under 400× magnification.

(1) Count the number of leukocytes seen per field within the monolayer of the smear.
(2) Count 10 fields and calculate the average number of cells seen per field.

$$\text{Average} \times 1.5 = \underline{\quad} \times 10^3/\mu L$$

Sources of error
- Poorly made smear
- Counting in areas too thick or too thin (see Figure 2.19).

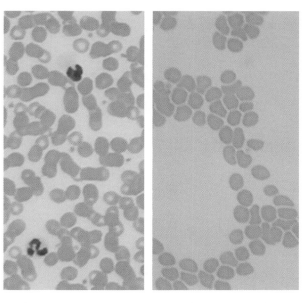

Figure 2.19   Area of the smear that is too thick (left) and too thin (right).

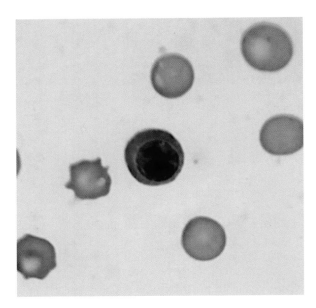

Figure 2.20   Nucleated red blood cell or NRBC.

Corrected white blood cell count

Purpose

Nucleated RBCs, or NRBCs (see Figure 2.20), can be seen in cases of regenerative anemia and in some bone marrow disorders. NRBCs can alter the accuracy of your WBC count. This is because they are a nucleated cell (like a WBC), and are mistakenly recorded as such by the analyzer. This results in a falsely high WBC count.

Performing a corrected white blood count adjusts your WBC count to account for these NRBCs.

Materials required

- Stained blood smear
- Microscope with 100× (oil immersion) objective lens
- Cell counter.

Procedure

NRBCs are first noted during your slide evaluation, usually while performing a WBC differential count.

(1) During your 100 cell differential count, record the number of NRBC seen.
(2) *Note*: Do not include NRBCs as a part of your 100 cell WBC differential. Record them separately.

$$\frac{100}{(100 + \text{No. of NRBC})} \times \text{WBC Count} \ (10^3/\mu L) = \_\_\_ \times 10^3/\mu L$$

Platelet count

Materials required
- Whole blood
- Thrombo-TIC test kit (Bioanalytic GmbH)
- Improved Neubauer hemocytometer
- Coverslip
- Microscope with 40× objective lens
- Cell counter.

Procedure
(1) Follow Thrombo-TIC instructions for proper filling of the vial.
(2) Place a clean coverslip on top of the hemocytometer.
(3) Mix the Thrombo-TIC vial, and flood one side of the hemocytometer counting chamber using capillary action.
(4) Count the platelets within 25 group squares (each consisting of 16 smallest squares) (see Figure 2.21).
(5) Repeat this count on the second side of the hemocytometer.
    Counts should not be done if platelet clumping is seen. If clumping is noted, repeat the dilution or collect a new blood sample if clumping persists.
(6) Calculate the sum of the 25 group squares for Side 1 and repeat for Side 2 of the hemocytometer grid.

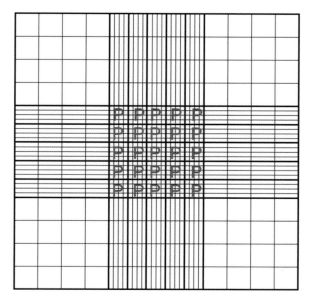

Figure 2.21   Platelet counting area, indicated by "P."

Calculations and quality control

Calculations should be made using the average between Side 1 and Side 2.

QC: Side 1 and Side 2 totals should be within 10% of each other before taking the average.

$$Average = \_\_\_ \times 10^3/\mu L$$

Sources of error

- Improper mixing of whole blood or prepared solution
- Improper filling of Thrombo-TIC vial
- Incomplete flooding or overfilling of the hemocytometer chamber
- Using a dirty hemocytometer can cause difficulty with differentiating between platelets and debris
- Platelet clumping present due to collection and/or handling of the blood sample.

Platelet estimate

Purpose

Performing a platelet estimate is a quick and simple way to verify adequate platelet numbers in a patient's sample. It is also useful when errors and flags arise during automated analysis of blood. Depending upon the analyzer, megathrombocytes, which are large platelets (see Figure 2.22), and platelet clumping can cause false readings.

Materials required

- Stained PBS
- Microscope with 100× objective lens
- Cell counter

Procedure

(1) First, scan the edges of the smear under low power for platelet clumps.

Because clumps are larger than individual cells, they will be pushed to the outer edges of the smear.

Tip: Platelet clumping is a common occurrence following the collection of blood from cats and horses. To avoid clumping, make a blood smear using fresh blood immediately following collection, before any anticoagulant is added.

If no clumping is seen, proceed with the estimate.

(2) Examine a stained blood smear under 1000× magnification.
(3) Count the number of platelets seen per field within the monolayer of the smear.
(4) Count 10 fields and calculate the average number of cells seen per field.

$$Average \times 20 = \_\_\_ \times 10^3/\mu L$$

Sources of error

- Poorly made smear
- Counting in areas too thick or too thin
- Platelet clumping present (see Figure 2.23).

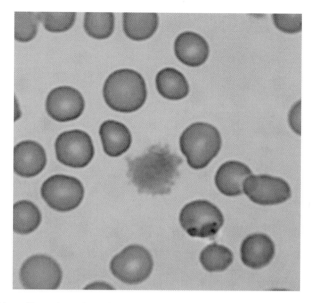

Figure 2.22   Megathrombocyte (giant platelet) (1000× magnification).

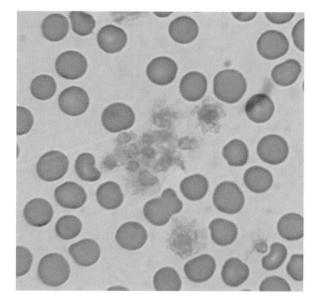

Figure 2.23   Platelet clumping (1000× magnification).

Normal species variation of leukocytes

Table 2.4   Canine leukocyte morphology.

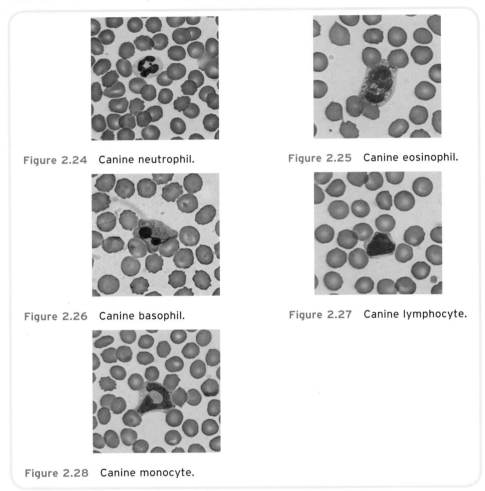

Figure 2.24   Canine neutrophil.

Figure 2.25   Canine eosinophil.

Figure 2.26   Canine basophil.

Figure 2.27   Canine lymphocyte.

Figure 2.28   Canine monocyte.

Note "teardrop"-shaped Barr body on the nucleus of a canine neutrophil (Figure 2.24). Occurs in females only.

Table 2.5   Feline leukocyte morphology.

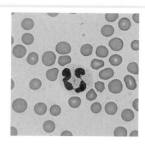

Figure 2.29   Feline neutrophil.

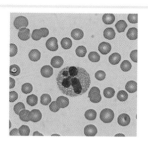

Figure 2.30   Feline eosinophil.

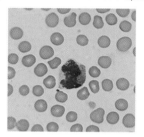

Figure 2.31   Feline basophil.

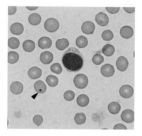

Figure 2.32   Feline lymphocyte.

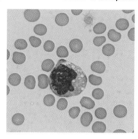

Figure 2.33   Feline monocyte.

Note the Howell-Jolly body (arrowhead) present in the red blood cell adjacent to the lymphocyte (Figure 2.32).

Table 2.6   Equine leukocyte morphology.

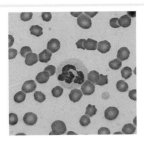

Figure 2.34   Equine neutrophil.

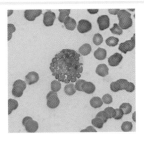

Figure 2.35   Equine eosinophil.

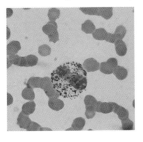

Figure 2.36   Equine basophil.

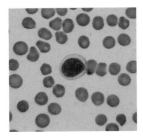

Figure 2.37   Equine lymphocyte.

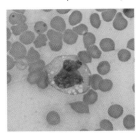

Figure 2.38   Equine monocyte.

Table 2.7   Bovine leukocyte morphology.

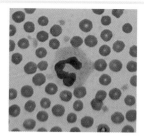

Figure 2.39   Bovine neutrophil.

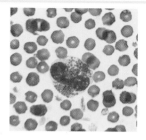

Figure 2.40   Bovine eosinophil.

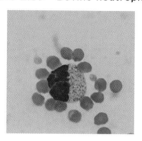

Figure 2.41   Bovine basophil.

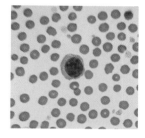

Figure 2.42   Bovine lymphocyte.

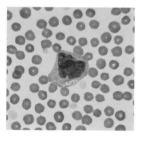

Figure 2.43   Bovine monocyte.

Table 2.8   Ovine leukocyte morphology.

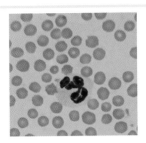

Figure 2.44   Ovine neutrophil.

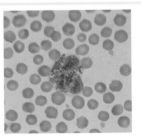

Figure 2.45   Ovine eosinophil.

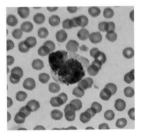

Figure 2.46   Ovine basophil.

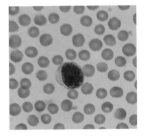

Figure 2.47   Ovine lymphocyte.

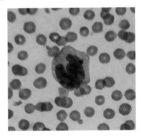

Figure 2.48   Ovine monocyte.

Neutrophil maturation

Table 2.9   The neutrophil in various stages of maturation. (Youngest to oldest, left to right.)

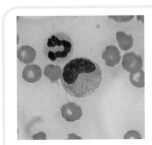

Figure 2.49
Metamyelocyte.

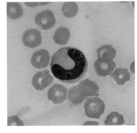

Figure 2.50   Band
neutrophil.

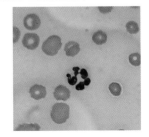

Figure 2.51   Hypersegmented
neutrophil.

Abnormal morphological changes in leukocytes

Table 2.10   Abnormal leukocyte morphology.

Toxic neutrophil	Cytoplasmic basophilia and vacuolation; Dohle bodies <ul><li>Associated with increased neutrophil production and shortened maturation time.</li></ul>	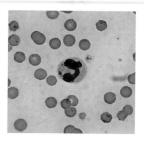 Figure 2.52 Toxic neutrophil. Note Dohle body present in the cytoplasm.
Atypical lymphocyte	Azurophilic cytoplasmic granules seen. <ul><li>Associated with chronic antigenic stimulation.</li></ul>	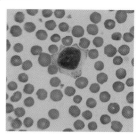 Figure 2.53 Atypical lymphocyte.
Reactive lymphocyte	Increased cytoplasmic basophilia is seen. <ul><li>Associated with antigenic stimulation secondary to vaccines or infection.</li></ul>	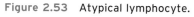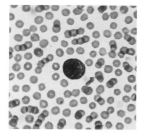 Figure 2.54 Reactive lymphocyte.

Erythrocyte morphologies

Table 2.11   Variations in erythrocyte chromasia (color).

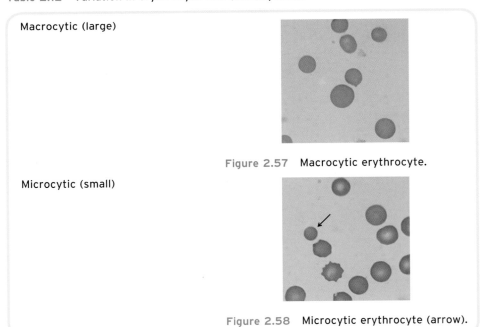

Hypochromic (pale)

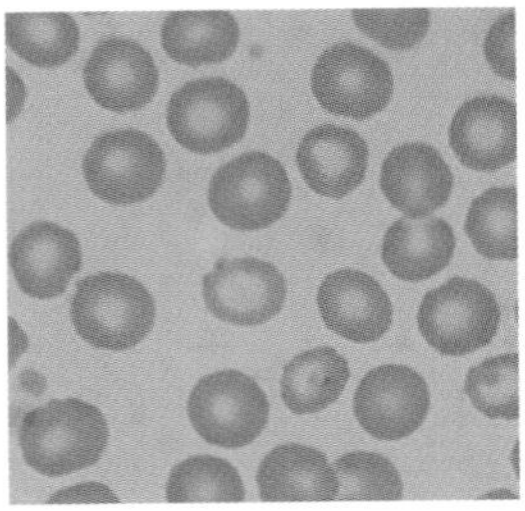

Figure 2.55   Hypochromic erythrocyte.

Polychromic (bluish)

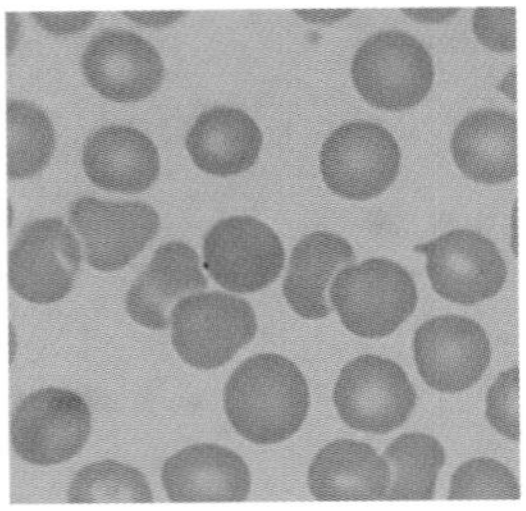

Figure 2.56   Polychromic erythrocyte.

Table 2.12   Variation in erythrocyte size (anisocytosis).

Macrocytic (large)

Figure 2.57   Macrocytic erythrocyte.

Microcytic (small)

Figure 2.58   Microcytic erythrocyte (arrow).

Table 2.13 Erythrocyte inclusion bodies.

Basophilic stippling

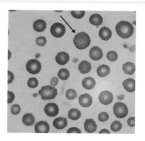

Figure 2.59   Basophilic stippling.

Howell–Jolly bodies

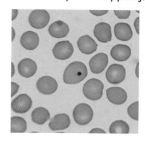

Figure 2.60   Howell-Jolly body.

Heinz bodies
(Diff-Quik stain)

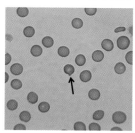

Figure 2.61   Heinz body (Diff-Quick stain).

Heinz bodies (new
methylene blue stain)

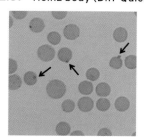

Figure 2.62   Heinz body (new methylene
blue stain).

Table 2.14   Small animal hemoparasites.

Babesia canis and *Babesia gibsoni*	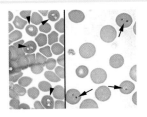 Figure 2.63 *Babesia canis* (left) and *Babesia gibsoni* (right) present on a canine blood film (from Thrall, Mary Anna, Weiser, Glade, Allison, Robin W., and Campbell, Terry W. 2012. *Veterinary Hematology and Clinical Chemistry*, 2nd ed. Ames: Blackwell Publishing).
Cytauxzoan	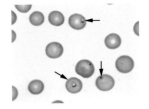 Figure 2.64 *Cytauxzoan* organisms on a feline blood film (from Thrall, Mary Anna, Weiser, Glade, Allison, Robin W., and Campbell, Terry W. 2012. *Veterinary Hematology and Clinical Chemistry*, 2nd ed. Ames: Blackwell Publishing).
Mycoplasma haemofelis (Figure 2.65) and *Mycoplasma haemocanis* (not shown)	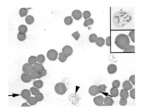 Figure 2.65 *Mycoplasma haemofelis* organisms appear as small, ring-shaped or rod-shaped structures. Organisms can be found on the surface or the edge of erythrocytes. Organisms also seen on the surface of "ghost" cells (arrowhead) (from Thrall, Mary Anna, Weiser, Glade, Allison, Robin W., and Campbell, Terry W. 2012. *Veterinary Hematology and Clinical Chemistry*, 2nd ed. Ames: Blackwell Publishing).

Table 2.15 Erythrocyte poikilocytosis (shape).

Dacrocyte

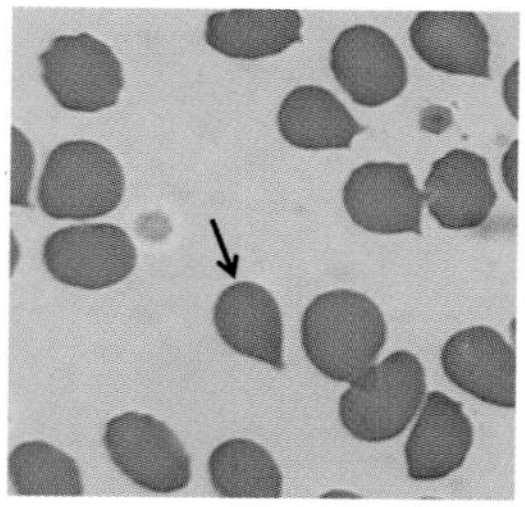

Figure 2.66 Dacrocyte.

Echinocyte

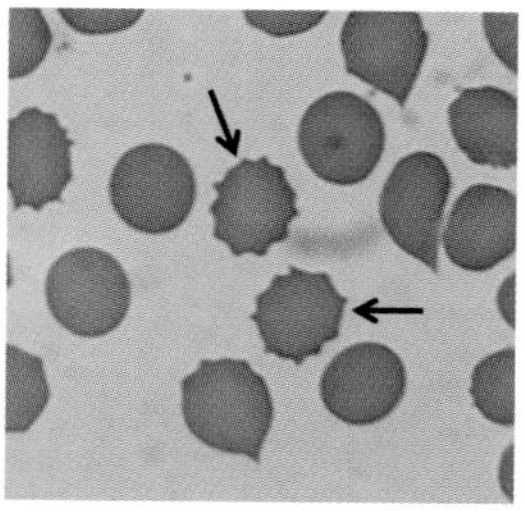

Figure 2.67 Echinocyte.

Schistocyte

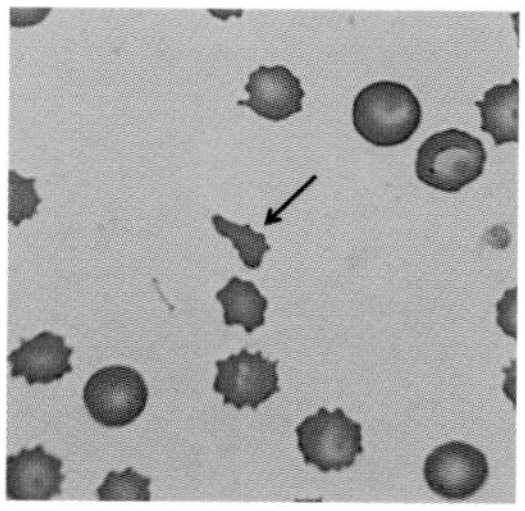

Figure 2.68 Schistocyte.

(Continued)

Table 2.15 (*Continued*)

Acanthocyte

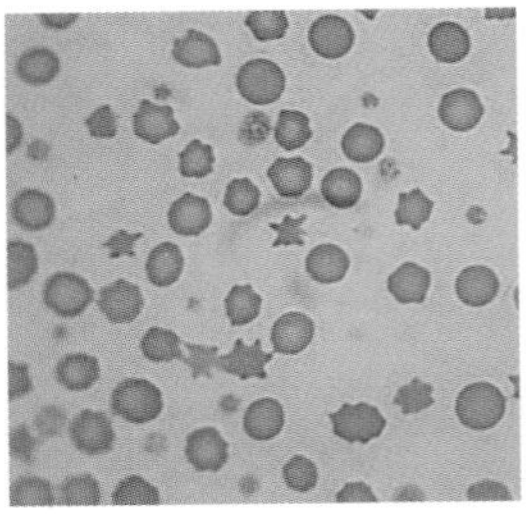

Figure 2.69   Acanthocyte.

Spherocyte

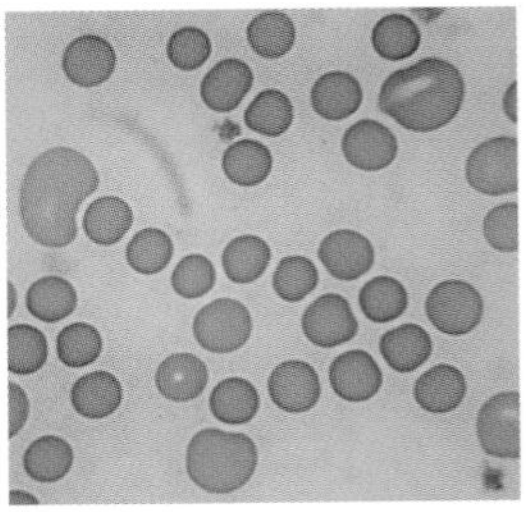

Figure 2.70   Spherocyte.

Keratocyte

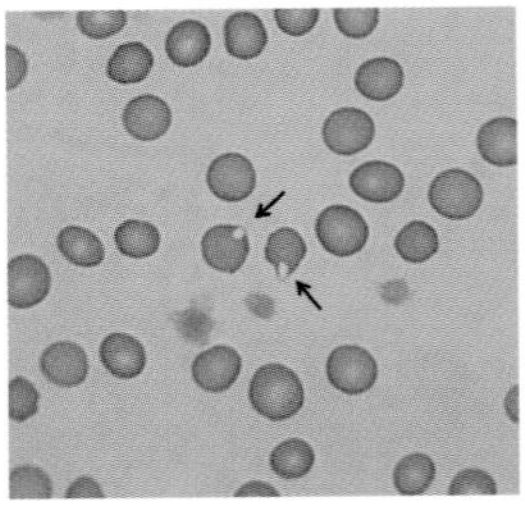

Figure 2.71   Keratocyte.

Codocyte

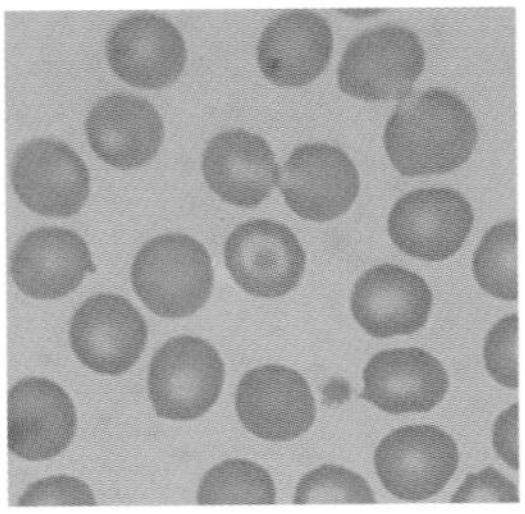

Figure 2.72   Codocyte.

Table 2.15 (Continued)

Stomatocyte

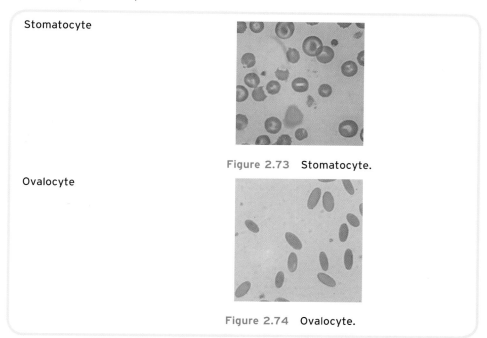

Figure 2.73 Stomatocyte.

Ovalocyte

Figure 2.74 Ovalocyte.

Evaluating a blood film to complement automated analyzers

Automated analyzers are a fast and convenient way to evaluate a patient's blood values. With this being said, analyzers should not completely eliminate the need to visually examine the blood smear microscopically. Microscopic examination accomplishes two important things: (1) you can confirm automated data, and (2) it allows you to evaluate the morphology of the blood cells. Performing a manual examination does not have to take much time, and the more often it is performed, the more proficient a technician will become.

Erythrocytes

Under 1000× magnification, examine the erythrocytes for their size and color. This will help to confirm the MCV and MCHC values calculated by the automated analyzer. A large variation in anisocytosis should be reflected in the analyzer's RDW (red cell distribution width) value. Increased numbers of polychromatophils can suggest an increased reticulocyte count and should be confirmed with a manual reticulocyte count if your analyzer is unable to perform this function. In addition, examine the erythrocytes for abnormal morphological characteristics and parasitic/infectious inclusions. Currently, no analyzer has the ability to evaluate these properties.

Leukocytes

Examining the numbers and distribution of the leukocytes will confirm the analyzers WBC count. Finally, examine the morphology of the leukocytes. Morphologies should be examined under 1000× magnification. Examine for the presence of band neutrophils, signs of toxicity, or other abnormal leukocytes. This could give insight to the presence and severity of an inflammatory response.

Thrombocytes

Thrombocytes are the most likely cell to cause problems for automated analyzers. This is largely in part to their tendency to clump. Examine your blood smear under 1000× magnification in the feathered edge for platelet clumping. Platelets sequestered into clumps will result in a low platelet count reading on the automated analyzer. Typically, a normal canine sample should have 10-35 platelets/1000× field.

The presence of large platelets, or megathrombocytes, is a typical finding in cats, but can suggest a bone marrow response in other species.

Tips for evaluating PBS

Perform a smear evaluation on *all* samples to complement the analyzer's readings—not only when abnormal results are given or when flags or errors are seen. It is of great value for a technician to familiarize themselves with what is considered "normal." Once this is achieved, "abnormal" morphologies or abnormal counts will be instantly obvious and more quickly identified, resulting in the entire process being accomplished more efficiently.

Clinical chemistries

To evaluate the function of most body systems, serum and/or plasma is evaluated for certain chemicals, enzymes, and compounds to show how the organs are performing. Chemistries (often called panels, databases, or profiles) are most frequently conducted on an in-house analyzer or sent to a reference laboratory. These chemistries reveal the level of the compound in the blood of the patient in comparison with the normal reference range for that species. Below is a list of the most routinely conducted chemistries and the organ or system they are associated with:

Table 2.16 Common clinical chemistry tests and their associated body system or organ.

Chemistry (and common abbreviation)	Body system or organ
Glucose (Glu, BG)	Required for every cell in the body—energy source
Urea nitrogen (BUN)	Kidney
Creatinine (Creat)	Kidney (waste product produced by the muscle)
	(Continued)

Table 2.16 (*Continued*)

Chemistry (and common abbreviation)	Body system or organ
Total protein (TP, TS)	Proteins in fluid portion of blood–albumin, globulin and others
Albumin (Alb)	Protein in blood, produced by the liver
Globulin (Gb, Glb)	Protein in blood associated with the immune system
Bilirubin, total (TBil, Total Bili, TB)	Liver (waste product from breakdown of RBC)
Alkaline phosphatase (Alk phos, ALP)	Liver and bone
Aspartate aminotransferase (AST, SGOT)	Liver (also found in heart)
Alanine aminotransferase (ALT, SGPT)	Most commonly associated with the liver (also found in kidney)
Calcium (Ca, Ca^{2+})	Mineral for muscles, nerves, heart, clotting and bones
Phosphorus (Phos, P, Ph)	Kidney, liver and bone
Sodium (Na, Na^+)	Electrolyte for normal processes in cells
Potassium (K, K^+)	Electrolyte for metabolism in cells
Chloride (Cl, Cl^-)	Electrolyte for acid-base balance in cells
Bicarbonate (CO_2)	Electrolyte for acid-base balance in cells
Amylase (Amyl, Amy)	Pancreas
Lipase (Lip)	Pancreas and upper GI
Creatine phosphokinase (CK, CPK)	Enzyme for heart, brain and skeletal muscle
Thyroid panel (T_4, Free T_4, TSH)	Thyroid function

Typically, the veterinarian will decide which combination of tests will be run based on the presenting complaint from the owner and the physical exam findings. Because testing procedures vary widely between analyzers and reference labs, they will not be covered.

Coagulation testing

In certain situations, animals require coagulation testing to determine if the clotting factors and platelets are working properly. Normal clotting function is a complex process (clotting/coagulation cascade) and requires many compounds and steps to achieve proper coagulation. Testing requires specific steps and can be highly technique sensitive. The most experienced technician should perform these tests. The jugular vein should be avoided as the collection vessel for any patients with a suspected coagulopathy, and a bandage should be applied to the venipuncture site.

Activated clotting time

Purpose
An activated clotting time (ACT) is an in-house test that is used to determine how portions (clotting factors) of the clotting cascade are working. The ACT will be prolonged in patients with faulty clotting factors and a low platelet count. Automated analyzers are becoming more common, making this test obsolete.

Materials required
- ACT tube (gray top)
- Vacutainer
- Warm water bath (body temperature of the species you are testing)
- Timer.

Procedure
(1) Perform a "clean" stick into the vein without poking or searching for the vessel. This will increase clotting factors and platelets erroneously.
(2) Allow the tube to fill to the volume according to the manufacturer.
(3) Begin gently mixing as soon as the collection is complete.
(4) Hold the tube in the water bath for 60 seconds then look for a clot. Then repeat every 5 seconds until a noticeable clot has formed. Do not shake or invert the tube during these repeated dips in the water other than carefully tilting to observe for a clot. Clotting times vary by species; however, a dog's blood should clot within 120 seconds and a cat's within 90 seconds.

Buccal mucosal bleeding time

Purpose
The buccal mucosal bleeding time (BMBT) test is used to determine primary hemostasis evaluating platelet numbers and function. It is typically used in patients with normal platelet numbers but questionable platelet function. This can also be used to diagnose von Willebrand disease seen primarily in Dobermans.

Materials required
- Gauze to tie the lips of the muzzle upward
- BMBT lancet (only a specific lancet for this test should be used; other devices will cause too deep of an incision)
- Filter paper or once-folded paper towel
- Timer.

Procedure

(1) Tie the muzzle of the dog closed with gauze with the lips turned upward. Cats and other species will likely need sedation.

(2) Utilizing the lancet, make a small, uniform incision on the underside of the lip. Bleeding will occur.

(3) Gently dab blood that flows from the incision with the paper. DO NOT touch the paper to the incision but just below so it collects the oozing blood.

(4) Time how long it takes for no more drips of blood to form at the incision. Dogs <4 minutes, cats <3.5 minutes.

Important notes

The muzzle should not be tied too tightly with the gauze as tissue damage could occur if left in place too long.

Automated clotting tests

Purpose

Many reference laboratories and in-house analyzers can perform tests to establish if clotting issues are present. A blue top tube is collected and analyzed for activated partial thromboplastin time (pTT, apTT), prothrombin time (PT), and thrombin time (TT). These three factors provide information on which portion of the clotting cascade may or may not be working properly.

Definitions

- **Activated partial thromboplastin time:** Measures the intrinsic factors and common pathways of the cascade.
- **Prothrombin time:** Measures the extrinsic factors and common pathways of the cascade.
- **Thrombin time:** Measures the functional activity of the final common pathway, namely fibrinogen.

An in-depth discussion of the clotting cascade is beyond the scope of this book; however, this section is meant to provide a basic understanding of coagulation tests, along with how and why they are performed.

Chapter 3
Urinalysis

Sample collection

The method in which a urine sample is obtained is very important to the interpretation of the urinalysis itself. The method of collection should *always* be noted on the urinalysis requisition at the time of analysis.

Free catch (voided sample)

Free catch samples are the easiest to collect and are often brought in by owners. They are an adequate sample for routine urinalysis, but are not appropriate for bacterial culturing. Owners can be instructed on how to collect samples at home in a manner that still maintains adequate quality control. A midstream, first-morning collection will provide the best sample for analysis (see Table 3.1).

Materials required
- Collection cup or ladle
- Pie plate or shallow dish (useful for female dogs)
- Nonabsorbent litter for collections in cats
- Specimen container

Good container choice for owners
- Leak proof with a tight-fitting lid
- Opaque
- Clean, and well rinsed of any previous contents or detergents
    Note the type of container the sample was collected in. For example, a butter container will have residue present that can cause microscopic lipid molecule contamination. This can lead to erroneous interpretations.
- For cats: Commercial nonabsorbent litter for urine collection is available. As a substitute, well-rinsed aquarium gravel or Styrofoam chips can be used as well.

Bladder expression

In small animals, bladder expression can be performed if a free catch sample is not possible. Like free catch samples, this collection method provides an adequate sample for routine urinalysis, but is not appropriate for bacterial culturing (see Table 3.2).

Veterinary Technician's Handbook of Laboratory Procedures, First Edition. Brianne Bellwood and Melissa Andrasik-Catton.
© 2014 John Wiley & Sons, Inc. Published 2014 by John Wiley & Sons, Inc.

Table 3.1 Advantages and disadvantages of a free catch (voided) sample.

Free catch (voided sample)

Advantages
- No risk or complications to the patient.
- Can be used by the client.

Disadvantages
- High amount of contamination of cells, bacteria and debris from the genitourinary tract, surrounding fur and the environment.
- Sample is unsuitable for culture.

Table 3.2 Advantages and disadvantages of bladder expression.

Bladder expression

Advantages
- Decreased risk of trauma (if done correctly).
- Sample can be obtained when needed.

Disadvantages
- Excessive pressure can result in trauma to the patient.
- If the bladder does not contain sufficient quantities of urine at the time, expression may not be successful.
- Same amount of contamination seen as with a voided sample.
- Sample is unsuitable for culture.

For collection, the animal is standing or placed in lateral recumbancy, and the bladder is palpated. Once it is located, gentle, steady pressure is applied to the bladder until the animal begins to urinate. It is important not to apply too much pressure as bladder rupture may occur. This method should *never* be used in patients with suspected obstruction or fragile bladders due to increased risk of rupture.

Materials required
- Collection dish
- Assistance with restraint

Catheterization

Catheterization involves inserting a rubber catheter into the urethra and feeding it up to the bladder of the patient to collect a sample. A sterile syringe is attached to the end of the catheter and urine is drawn out. This procedure varies slightly depending upon species and sex. In any case, sterility is important. Sterile catheters, sterile lubricant, and sterile gloves should be worn to prevent infection. For female animals, a speculum may be used to ease visualization of the urethral opening. Samples collected by this method in a sterile manner may be suitable for bacterial culturing (see Table 3.3).

Table 3.3   Advantages and disadvantages of catheterization.

Advantages
• Sample is collected in a sterile manner; therefore, it is suitable for culture.
• Can collect urine sample when bladder volume is low.

Disadvantages
• Increased risk of an iatrogenic infection or trauma.
• Difficult to perform in female animals.

Materials required
• Sterile polypropylene or rubber catheter
• Sterile lubricant
• Sterile gloves
• Sterile syringe for collection
• Speculum (for female patients).

Cystocentesis

Cystocentesis is another method for collecting a sterile urine sample, and therefore is appropriate for bacterial culture. The procedure should only be performed on quiet, easily restrained animals. Sedation may be required to achieve this. Typically, the patient is restrained in dorsal recumbancy and the bladder is palpated. An ultrasound may also be used to visualize the bladder and help guide the needle. The site should be cleaned with 70% alcohol and aseptic techniques should be followed. A 1″–1 1/2″, 25–22 gauge needle, attached to a syringe, is inserted through the abdominal wall and into the bladder. Once inserted, the needle is never redirected as this could cause potential damage to adjacent organs. With the needle in the bladder, the plunger on the syringe is retracted and urine is drawn out. Once the sample has been obtained, the negative pressure on the syringe should be released before the needle is removed. For female dogs and cats, the needle is inserted along the midline of the caudal abdomen. For male dogs, the needle is inserted caudal to the umbilicus, just off to the side of the sheath (see Table 3.4).

Materials required
• 1″–1.5″, 25–22 gauge needle
• 10–12 mL syringe
• Assistance with restraint.

Sample preservation

Fresh urine should be examined within 20 minutes of collection. If that is not possible, then a method of preservation should be considered.

Table 3.4 Advantages and disadvantages of cystocentesis.

Advantages
- Less of a risk of causing an iatrogenic infection (compared with catheterization).
- No contamination of urine; therefore, the sample is suitable for culture.

Disadvantages
- Requires adequate volume of urine within the bladder.
- May cause microscopic hematuria.

Before choosing a preservative, consider the following:

(1) The method of sample collection used
(2) The analyses to be performed
(3) The biochemical method that will be used
(4) The time delay between urine collection and analysis.

Note: **Always indicate the type of preservative used on the requisition.**

In vitro changes occurring in unpreserved urine

Physical characteristics
Turbidity: Increase—as bacteria, and possibly crystals, multiply, the turbidity of the sample increases.
Odor: Becomes stronger smelling, as microbes cause increased amounts of ammonia to be produced within the sample.

Chemical characteristics
pH: Increase or decrease—depending upon the types of microbes present in the sample.
Glucose: Decrease—as it is metabolized by cells and microbes.
Ketones: Decrease—being a volatile substance, ketones evaporate from the sample.
Bilirubin: Decrease—bilirubin levels decrease in the presence of direct light.
Nitrite: Increase—if it is produced by the types of microbes present in the sample.

Sediment characteristics
Cellular structures: Decrease—cells begin to deteriorate in concentrated, dilute, or acidic urine.
Crystals: Increase or decrease—depending on the solubility and pH of the sample, the numbers of various crystals may change over time.
Bacteria: Increase—bacterial populations increase over time within the sample.

Refrigeration

Refrigerating a urine sample is an adequate form of preservation for up to 6 hours. Before analyzing the sample, be sure to allow it to return to room temperature first.

This is important for the enzymatic reactions that occur during the chemical examination of urine. Generally, enzymatic reactions occur at a slower rate when the sample is at a lower temperature. This results in false readings.

Lowering the temperature may also encourage crystal formation. As the sample returns to room temperature, these crystals will dissolve.

The accuracy of specific gravity (SG) readings on refractometers can also be compromised when analyzing a sample that is below room temperature.

Freezing

Preserving urine by freezing will inhibit bacterial growth, thus avoiding changes caused by the actions of microbes. Freezing is also adequate for most chemical tests and preserves the mineral content of urine. Freezing, however, is an unsuitable method of preservation for sediment and hormonal analyses due to the resulting cellular and protein damage.

Toluene

Toluene is an organic solvent that can be used to preserve a urine sample. Toluene floats on the surface of the sample, preventing the loss of acetone and contamination. Two milliliters of toluene will be adequate for 100 mL of urine. Toluene is suitable for preserving the chemical profile of the urine sample; however, it would not prevent the *in vitro* growth of microbes present in the sample. Due to the fact that toluene is a solvent, care should be taken in choosing an appropriate container in which to preserve the urine.

Formalin (40%)

One drop of 40% formalin added to 30 mL of urine is adequate to preserve the sample for sediment analysis. Formalin prevents microbial growth, therefore preserving the cellular integrity of various structures within the sample. Formalin is a reducing agent, so it does interfere with the chemical analysis of substances that use this principle in their enzymatic reactions. One example is glucose determination using reagent strips. The use of enough formalin can result in a false negative.

Boric acid (0.8%)

The addition of boric acid to a sample will inhibit bacterial growth. Boric acid is an appropriate preservative for sediment analysis and, with the exception of pH, chemical analysis as well.

Commercial preservation tablets

Commercial preservation tablets are designed to inhibit microbes and control the pH of a urine sample, usually for a period of up to 5 days. They also provide good preservation of urine sediment, such as leukocytes, erythrocytes, casts, and crystals.

Physical examination of urine

The physical examination of urine consists of assessing the volume, color, turbidity, odor, and SG of a urine sample.

Volume

An accurate representation of urine volume should be assessed over a period of 24 hours. All voided urine is collected and measured to determine if the quantity produced is appropriate. When assessing urine volume, ensure consistency with the patient's regular routine. (i.e., regular diet and access to water; regular medications and/or supplements). Normal daily urine output can be calculated using a rate of 1mL/kg/h.

Terminology related to urine volume
Polyuria: Increased amounts of urine volume
Oliguria: Decreased amounts of urine volume
Anuria: No urine production.

Color

Normal urine is described as being straw colored. The pigment of the urine often correlates with the concentration of the sample, but this should still be confirmed with a SG reading.

To avoid discrepancies among technicians, use standard color terms when recording your findings (see Table 3.5 and Figure 3.1).

Table 3.5 Common urine colors and associated causes.

Straw	Normal
Colorless-pale	Dilute urine
Deep yellow	Concentrated urine; bilirubinuria
Orange-red	Hematuria; hemoglobinuria
Red-brown	Myoglobinuria
Milky white	Pyuria

Turbidity

Turbidity refers to the "cloudiness" of urine. An increase in turbidity in the urine can be caused by cellular elements, crystals, microorganisms, or mucous. When examining the turbidity of a sample, there are a few key points to remember:

- Ensure your sample is well mixed by inverting the container several times prior to examination. Items listed above that can cause an increase in turbidity will settle to the bottom of a standing sample.
- Assess turbidity on a room temperature sample.

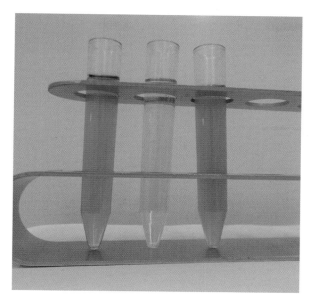

Figure 3.1   Urine color variations. From left to right: straw, pale yellow, and orange-red.

- Examine the turbidity in a clear container of a standard depth. A good choice is a urine tube or sterile red top blood collection tube.
- Horses and rabbits typically have turbid urine. This is due to the presence of mucous and calcium carbonate crystals. Turbid urine is considered normal in these species.

To examine turbidity:

(1) With the sample in a clear tube, invert several times to ensure the sample is well mixed.
(2) Hold the sample up in front of a piece of paper with text on it.
(3) Assess how clear the lettering can be viewed through the sample (see Figure 3.2).
(4) Record as clear (0), slightly cloudy (1), cloudy (2), or turbid (3).

Odor

The odor of urine can provide insight into possible conditions that should later be confirmed through chemical and sediment analysis.

Again, it is important to use standard terminology to minimize discrepancies among technicians:

Strong odor: The urine of intact male animals, especially cats and goats, is often quite strong and should be described as such.

Ammonia: Ammonia-scented urine can be associated with cystitis. Some species of bacteria metabolize urea in the urine to ammonia, producing a distinguishing odor.

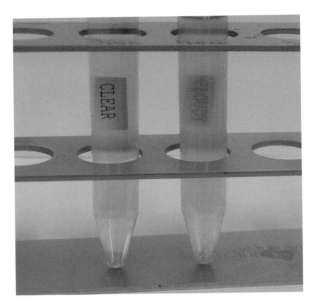

Figure 3.2   Assessing turbidity.

The presence of bacteria should be confirmed during the sediment examination or with a urine culture.

Putrid: Putrid- (or foul-) smelling urine is associated with the degradation of protein. This can occur during infections, and should be confirmed with further testing.

Fruity: Increased ketones present in the urine give off a fruity odor. This odor may also be noticed on the patient's breath when they are in a state of ketosis.

Specific gravity (SG)

SG is determined by assessing the density of a liquid (in this case, urine) compared with the density of distilled water.

Measuring SG requires the use of a refractometer (see Figure 3.3).

In a correctly calibrated refractometer, distilled water should read 1.000. Calibration should be checked regularly to ensure accuracy.

If the urine sample that is being tested exceeds the maximum limit of the refractometer, an accurate SG can be achieved by following these steps:

(1) Mix equal portions of urine with distilled water.
(2) Place a drop of this mixture on the refractometer and obtain the reading.
(3) Multiply the last two digits of the reading by 2 in order to obtain the estimated SG.

Terminology related to SG

Hypersthenuria: The SG of the urine is higher than the glomerular filtrate (dogs: >1.030; cats: >1.035).

Hyposthenuria: The SG of the urine is lower than the glomerular filtrate (<1.008).

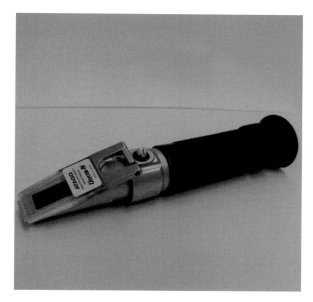

Figure 3.3   Refractometer.

Isosthenuria: The SG of the urine is equal to that of the glomerular filtrate (1.008–1.012).

Tips for accurate SG readings
● Ensure the sample is well mixed before reading.
● Ensure the sample is at room temperature if it was previously refrigerated.
● Practice good equipment maintenance.

Specific gravity readings using reagent strips
Many commercial reagent strips have a pad allotted to measuring the SG of a urine sample. This method of measurement differs from the refract meter method and has some significant drawbacks that make it unreliable for the veterinary practice.

(1) The principle of the test involves the use of a pH indicator to produce a degree of color change associated with a SG value. Urine samples with a pH of 6.5 or higher could result in erroneous findings.
(2) The highest SG reading the strip can measure is 1.030, which is below the capacity of dogs and cats.

Chemical examination

The chemical examination of urine is usually performed by the use of reagent strips. These are multiparameter strips that contain a number of pads, each designed to test

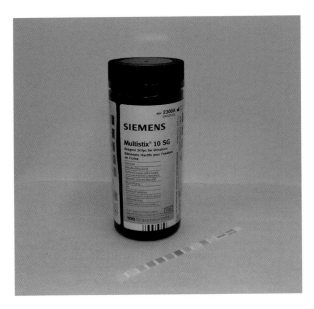

Figure 3.4 Multistix 10.

for a specific urine constituent. Commercial examples would be Multistix or Chemstrip (see Figure 3.4).

There are individual tests available that can be used as well. Depending upon the constituent tested, these alternative methods may be more/less specific or may simply be useful as a confirmatory test.

Whichever method is chosen, it is important to review the package insert and make note of the testing time required and any possible false positives or false negatives that can occur.

Glucose

The term used to describe glucose in the urine is glucosuria. The reagent strip method for detecting glucose is specific for glucose, meaning no other sugar will cause a positive result.

Possible causes of false positives with the reagent strips are contamination with hydrogen peroxide, as well as other strong oxidizing agents, such as chlorine. False negatives (or decreased values) can be seen in urine samples preserved with formalin.

Clinitest tablets are also available to detect glucose in the urine. These tablets will detect any sugar (or reducing substance) in the urine, and therefore are not specific to glucose.

Bilirubin

When bilirubin is present in the urine, the term "bilirubinuria" is used. Bilirubin is unstable in sunlight or artificial light and should therefore be tested immediately. Delaying testing will result in false negative values.

Ictotest tablets are available to test for the presence of bilirubin in a urine sample. Ictotest tablets are more sensitive than reagent strips and are able to detect smaller quantities of bilirubin.

Ketones

There are three ketone bodies that are produced: acetone, acetoacetic acid, and β-hydroxybutyric acid. Most reagent strips are sensitive to acetoacetic acid, less sensitive to acetone, and do not detect β-hydroxybutyric acid. The presence of ketone bodies in the urine, or ketonuria, is often accompanied by a fruity odor.

In addition to the reagent strips, individual tablet tests called Acetest are available. Acetest relies on the same testing principle as the reagent strips, but is more sensitive.

Blood

Reagent strips have the ability to detect intact RBC (hematuria), free hemoglobin (hemoglobinuria), and myoglobin (myoglobinuria) in a urine sample. The test is quite sensitive, and positive samples may appear normal in color during the physical exam.

Hematest tablets that were originally developed for detecting blood in feces can be used in urine samples; however, they are less sensitive than reagent strips.

To avoid false negatives, be sure to mix and resuspend the sample before testing. Certain microbes and cells, if present, can produce the enzyme peroxidase, which will result in a false positive. Another source of a false positive is contamination with oxidizing disinfectants.

pH

pH testing through reagent strips offer analysis of the urine's acidity or alkalinity over a pH range of 5.0-8.5. Results are read at 0.5 intervals on the pH scale. Care should be taken when using the reagent stick as not to contaminate the pH pad with the acidic buffer contained within the neighboring protein pad.

Protein

When protein is present in the urine, the term proteinuria is used. Reagent strips are not specific for any particular protein. They primarily detect albumin and are less sensitive for globulins and mucoproteins.

False negatives may occur due to the low concentration of protein contained within the sample. The concentration may fall below the sensitivity level of the reagent strip.

For the detection of microalbuminuria, certain in-house enzyme-linked immunosorbent assay (ELISA) test kits are able to detect the trace amounts of albumin that would be missed by the reagent strip method.

Urobilinogen

When testing for urobilinogen, the same light-sensitivity precautions used for bilirubin should be taken. Other false negatives can result from the use of formalin as a preservative.

Nitrite

Nitrites are products formed from nitrates by the actions of certain species of bacteria. Because of this, the presence of nitrites can suggest a bacterial infection, but the absence of nitrites should not rule it out. The reagent strips are specific for nitrites only, but there are several factors to consider when recording nitrite levels as negative. First, only certain species of bacteria will convert nitrate to nitrite. Second, it takes time for this to occur. A short urine retention time within the bladder may not be adequate for this conversion to take place.

Leukocytes

Leukocytes present in the urine are termed pyuria. The reagent strip method for detecting leukocytes relies on the detection of a leukocyte esterase enzyme. Unfortunately, this test is insensitive in dogs, and almost always gives a positive result for feline samples, regardless of the presence of leukocytes. The presence or absence of leukocytes should always be confirmed with a sediment examination.

Sediment examination

Sediment examination is the final step of a complete urinalysis. A sediment exam not only allows the technician to visualize structures such as cells, crystals, and casts, but it also serves to confirm suspected findings during the physical and chemical examinations previously conducted.

The SG of the sample itself can have an effect on the appearance of some structures, specifically leukocytes and erythrocytes. This is due to the process of osmosis. In samples with a SG >1.020, these cells will begin to appear smaller, distorted, and shriveled. In more dilute urine, (<1.010), the cells will swell and may eventually rupture if given enough time.

Before examining the sediment, we must first concentrate the sample. This is done by centrifuging the urine. After centrifugation, the urine will be separated into two portions: the supernatant and the sediment(see Figure 3.5).

Materials required

- Conical urine tubes
- Centrifuge
- Microscope
- Slides and cover slip
- Sediment stain (if preferred).

Sediment stain

Sediment stain can be a useful tool in the examination of urine. Many microscopic elements are translucent, and stain can provide some color or contrast to make visualization easier. If using stain, it is still a good practice to prepare one sample without stain and one with stain, then examine and compare both.

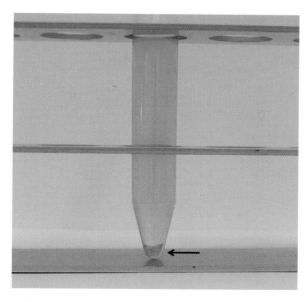

Figure 3.5   Urine after centrifugation. Sediment is concentrated at the bottom (arrow).

Stain can bring with it some undesirable findings as well. Older stain can precipitate, causing clumps which could obscure or interfere with your readings. Stain can also harbor bacteria and fungus, resulting in a possible false positive for bacteria in your microscopic examination. Comparing a stained sample with an unstained sample can help in eliminating these false positives.

To maintain good quality control, check your stain regularly. Examine the stain by adding one drop to a slide, add a coverslip, and view under 40× power. Scan the area for bacteria and stain precipitate. If these contaminants are found, discard the stain. Sediment stain is relatively inexpensive and should be routinely replaced on a monthly basis.

Procedure for microscopic examination of urine

(1) Pour 10 mL of the urine sample into a labeled conical centrifuge tube. If 10 mL is not available, note the volume used on your requisition.
(2) Centrifuge the sample for 5 minutes at 1500 rpm.
(3) Decant the supernatant leaving approximately 0.5–1 mL in the tube.
(4) Resuspend the sediment by flicking the tube with your fingers or gently mixing the sediment and supernatant with a pipette.
(5) Transfer a drop of resuspended sediment near the end of a microscope slide with a transfer pipette and place a coverslip over it.
(6) *Optional*: Add one drop of sediment stain to one drop of urine sediment on the other end of the microscope slide and place a coverslip over it.
(7) Increase the light contrast of the microscope by partially closing the iris diaphragm.

(8) Scan the entire slide under low power (10×) for the presence of large formed elements, such as casts, crystals, and clusters of cells.
(9) Using a grid pattern, examine the entire specimen under the coverslip (both stained and unstained samples)using high power (40×) to identify and semi-quantify formed elements.

Tip: To verify the presence of cellular components, make a blood smear with the sediment. Dry and stain with a Wright's type stain and examine microscopically.

Reporting of findings

Casts are examined and evaluated as the average number seen per low power (10×) field. Red blood cells and white blood cells are evaluated as the average number seen per high power field (40×). Other elements, such as bacteria and crystals, are also examined under high power (40×), and reported as occasional (1+), few (2+), moderate (3+), or many (4+).

Microscopic elements of urine sediment

Table 3.6   Cellular constituents of urine sediment.

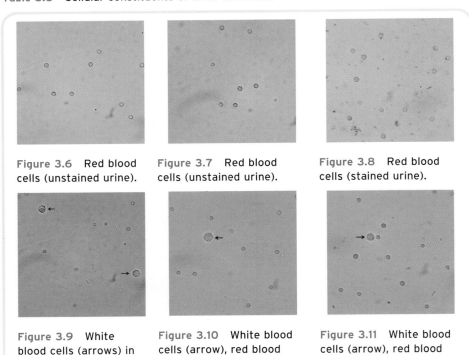

Figure 3.6   Red blood cells (unstained urine).

Figure 3.7   Red blood cells (unstained urine).

Figure 3.8   Red blood cells (stained urine).

Figure 3.9   White blood cells (arrows) in unstained urine. Red blood cells and bacteria are present as well.

Figure 3.10   White blood cells (arrow), red blood cells, and bacteria present in unstained urine.

Figure 3.11   White blood cells (arrow), red blood cells, and bacteria present in stained urine.

Table 3.6   (*Continued*)

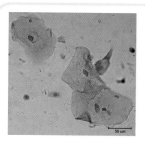

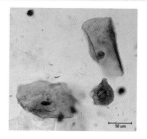

Figure 3.12 Squamous epithelial cell. Bacilli bacteria and WBCs are also present.

Figure 3.13 Two squamous epithelial cells, and one smaller, transitional epithelial cell.

Figure 3.14 Renal tubular cells.

Table 3.7   Urinary casts.

Hyaline cast

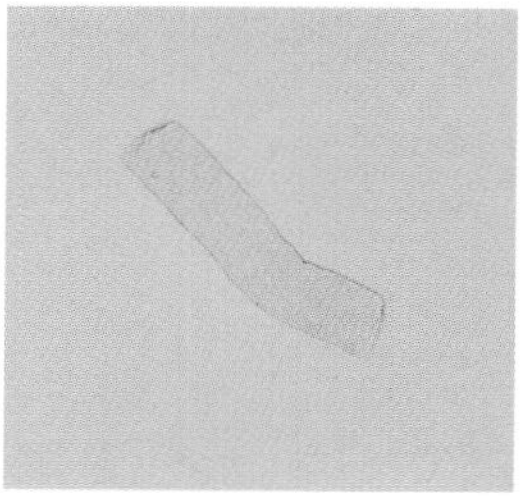

Figure 3.15 Hyaline cast (from Hendrix, Charles M. and Sirois, Margi. 2007. *Laboratory Procedures for Veterinary Technicians*, 5th ed. St. Louis: Mosby-Elsevier).

Epithelial cast

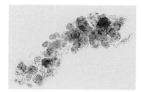

Figure 3.16 Epithelial cast (from Hendrix, Charles M. and Sirois, Margi. 2007. *Laboratory Procedures for Veterinary Technicians*, 5th ed. St. Louis: Mosby-Elsevier).

Granular cast

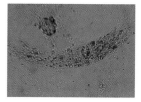

Figure 3.17 Granular cast (from Hendrix, Charles M. and Sirois, Margi. 2007. *Laboratory Procedures for Veterinary Technicians*, 5th ed. St. Louis: Mosby-Elsevier).

Table 3.8   Urinary crystals.

Type	pH	
Ammonium urate	Acidic/neutral	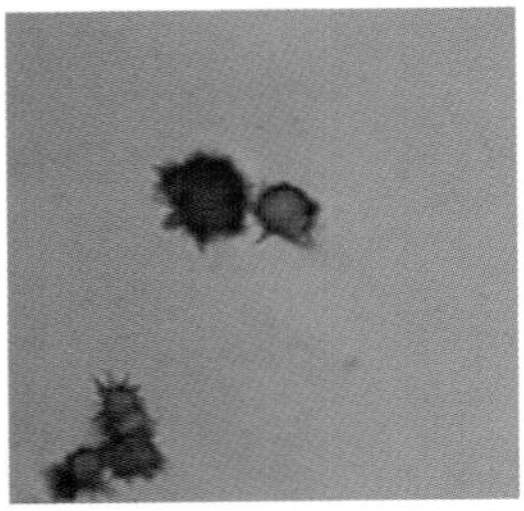 Figure 3.18 Ammonium urate crystals (from McCurnin, Dennis M. and Bassert, Joanna M. 2006. *Clinical Textbook for Veterinary Technicians*, 6th ed. St. Louis: Saunders-Elsevier).
Amorphous urate	Acidic/neutral	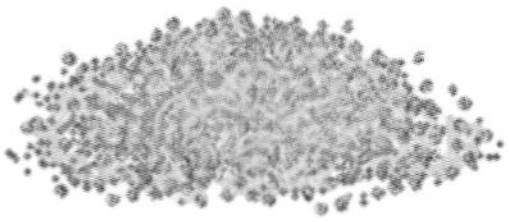 Figure 3.19 Amorphous urate crystals.
Bilirubin	Acidic	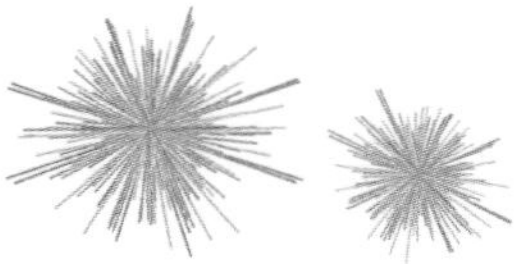 Figure 3.20 Bilirubin crystals.
Calcium carbonate	Neutral/alkaline	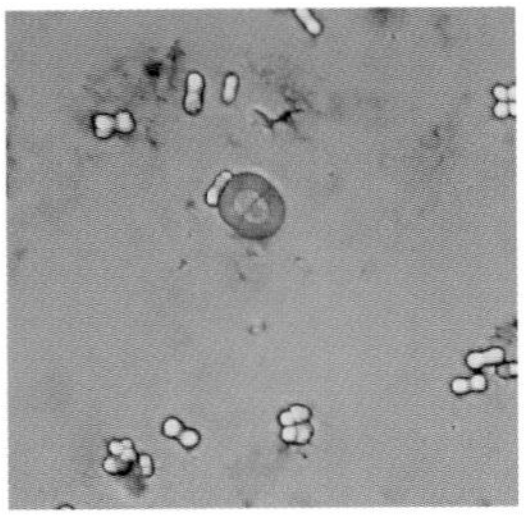 Figure 3.21 Calcium carbonate crystals (spherical and dumbbell forms) present in equine urine.

Table 3.8 (Continued)

Type	pH	
Calcium oxalate dihydrate	Acidic/neutral	

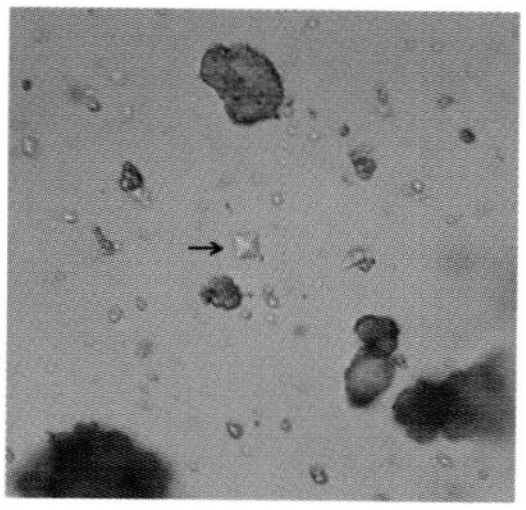

Figure 3.22 Calcium oxalate dihydrate crystals.

Calcium oxalate monohydrate	Acidic/neutral	

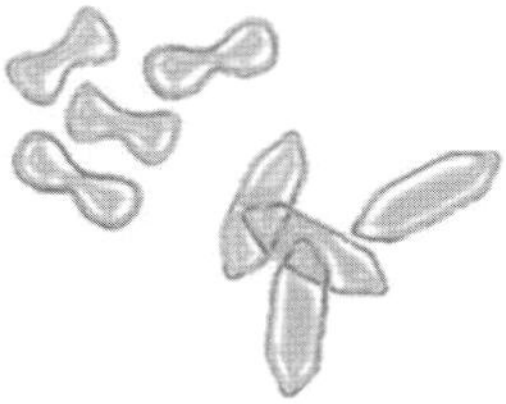

Figure 3.23 Calcium oxalate monohydrate.

Cholesterol	Acidic/neutral	

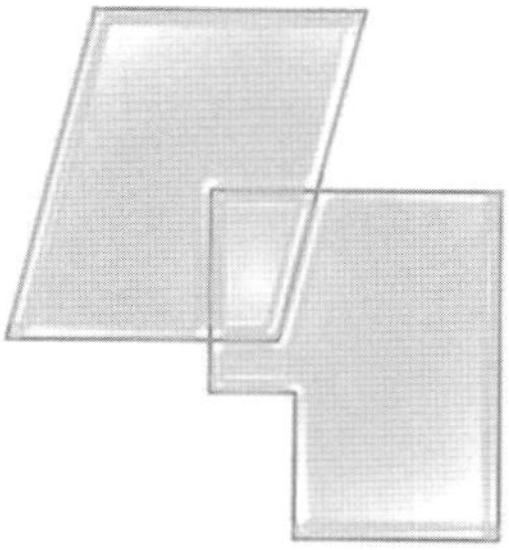

Figure 3.24 Cholesterol crystal.

(Continued)

Table 3.8   (Continued)

Type	pH
Cystine	Acidic/neutral

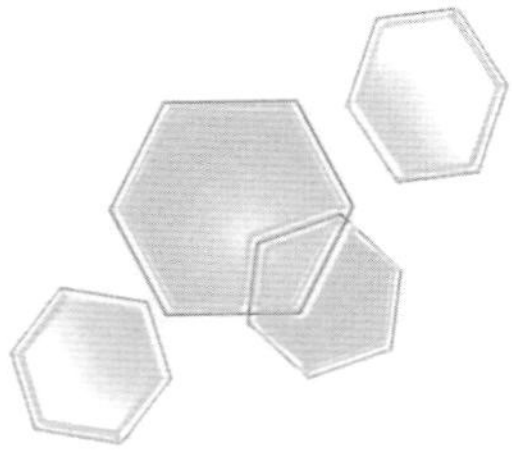

Figure 3.25   Cystine crystal.

Magnesium ammonium phosphate	Neutral/alkaline

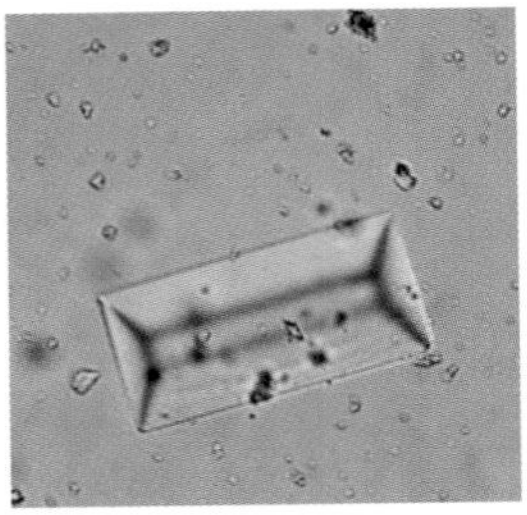

Figure 3.26   Magnesium ammonium phosphate (struvite) crystal.

Sulfa metabolite	Acidic/neutral

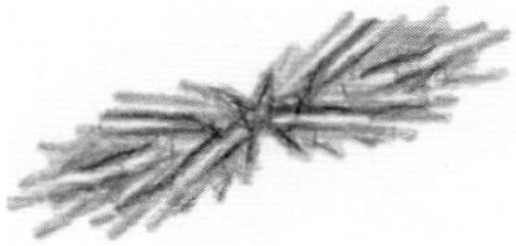

Figure 3.27   One form of sulfa metabolite crystal.

Table 3.9   Miscellaneous findings in urine sediment.

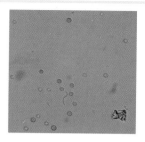

Figure 3.28   A chain of cocci bacteria present in a urine sample. Rod-shaped bacilli and RBCs are also present.

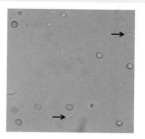

Figure 3.29   Bacilli bacteria (arrows) and RBCs also present.

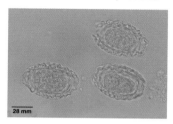

Figure 3.30   *Dioctophymarenale ovum* (from Zajac, Anne M. and Conboy, Gary A. 2012. *Veterinary Clinical Parasitology*, 8th ed. Ames: Blackwell Publishing).

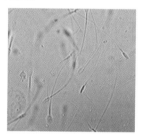

Figure 3.31   Spermatozoa.

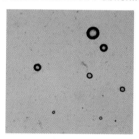

Figure 3.32   Artifact: bubbles.

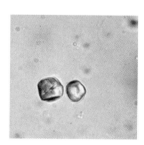

Figure 3.33   Starch granules.

Chapter 4
Parasitology

Collection

As in many other aspects of laboratory analysis, sample collection in parasitology is important in achieving accurate results.

In small animal medicine, fecal samples are often brought in by clients. These samples can certainly be acceptable if proper collection instructions are given to the owner ahead of time.

- The sample should be fresh. If samples cannot be examined within 2 hours, they should be refrigerated. As feces age, a diagnosis can be compromised, as eggs larvate and oocysts sporulate.
- Samples obtained later from the yard, pen, or litter box are *not* acceptable.
- The volume of sample should be adequate. A minimum of 10 g of fresh feces should be collected.

In large animal medicine, fecal samples are collected directly from an animal's rectum if possible. Store collected samples in proper fecal containers (see Figure 4.1), and avoid using OB sleeves as alternatives. OB sleeves are difficult to label properly and can be messy to retrieve a sample from for analysis.

Pooled samples

Pooled fecal samples describes a collection of fecal samples obtained from a group of animals that are housed together (e.g., feedlot cattle). In these instances, no one specific individual is identified, rather the sample represents the group. It is important to note that the results of this fecal analysis will result in the whole herd being treated for the parasite. When collecting these samples, the label should clearly state:

- Owner
- Date/time of collection
- Pen number
- Number of animals contained within this pen.

Veterinary Technician's Handbook of Laboratory Procedures, First Edition. Brianne Bellwood and Melissa Andrasik-Catton.
© 2014 John Wiley & Sons, Inc. Published 2014 by John Wiley & Sons, Inc.

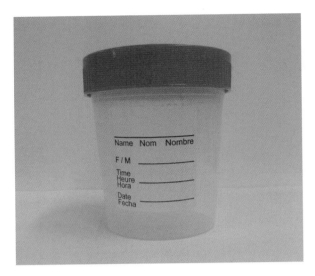

Figure 4.1 Specimen container suitable for fecal collection.

Gross examination

Upon receipt of a fecal sample, a gross exam should first be performed to examine the physical characteristics.

Consistency

Comment on the consistency of the fecal sample. Is it soft, watery, or hard? Keep in mind that "normal" consistency varies depending upon the species from which it came.

Color

Unusual color should be noted, as it could give insight into other underlying conditions, for example, gray stool can indicate pancreatic insufficiency.

Blood

Note any blood present. Blood may appear bright red (frank), or black (melena or melanous) and have a tar-like consistency.

Mucous

Mucous may be present on the surface of fresh feces. This should be noted.

Gross parasites

Parasites may be visible upon gross examination of the stool. Most commonly seen in dog or cat feces are roundworms and the proglotids of tapeworms.

Microscopic examination

There are many methods of preparing and performing a microscopic examination. The goal of each is to detect parasite ova or oocysts in the patient's sample. Depending upon the suspected parasite, the sample, or equipment available, one method may be preferred over another.

Regardless of the preparation method, the examination procedure should be consistent. Examine the entire coverslip, working in a methodical grid pattern to ensure everything is visualized. The examination should be performed initially using the 10× objective for scanning, and then 40× objective to further identify any ova present.

Direct fecal smear

One advantage to the direct smear method is that is requires very little feces. This technique can even be used on the small amount of fecal material found on the end of a thermometer. The downside to this technique is that with such a small sample, the chance of finding evidence of a parasite is greatly reduced.

Materials
- Microscope slides
- Coverslip
- Saline
- Wooden applicator stick

Procedure
(1) Using a wooden applicator stick, mix a small amount of fecal material into a few drops of saline in the center of a slide.
(2) Blend gently until the mixture is homogenous.
(3) Spread out the mixture to a thin layer.
(4) Remove any large fecal pieces.
(5) Place a coverslip over the sample (see Figure 4.2).
(6) Examine microscopically.

This technique is particularly useful for viewing live, motile, trophozoites (e.g., *Giardia*).

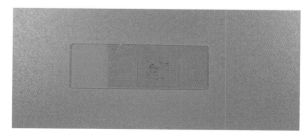

Figure 4.2   Mounted direct smear.

Simple fecal flotation

There are several types of fecal flotation solutions that are used as a semi-quantitative method of evaluating a fecal sample. In these methods, an estimate is made of the number of parasite ova per gram of feces.

The principle behind this method is to use the differences in specific gravity of parasite eggs and cysts from that of fecal debris and the solution. A fecal sample is mixed with a flotation solution consisting of various salts or sugars added to water to increase its specific gravity. Parasite eggs and cysts float to the surface, while most fecal matter sinks to the bottom.

A common flotation medium is sodium nitrate solution. It can be purchased already prepared and is used in diagnostic kits (see Figure 4.3).

Other popular solutions include Sheather's solution and zinc sulfate.

Sheather's solution, also known as sugar solution, can be messy to work with as it is quite sticky. It tends to float fewer eggs as compared with sodium nitrate, but it does not distort roundworm eggs. It is readily available and inexpensive.

Zinc sulfate does an excellent job in concentrating cystic forms of protozoans. Zinc sulfate is available from veterinary suppliers.

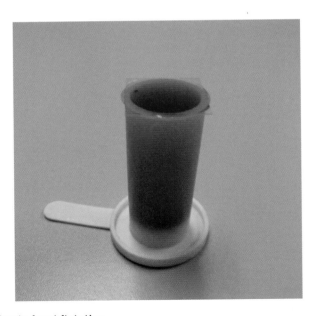

Figure 4.3 Simple fecal flotation.

Materials (commercially available fecal flotation kits may be used in place of these supplies)

- Two specimen containers (or wax paper cups)
- Tongue depressor
- Flotation solution
- Fecal shell vial (or test tube)
- Metal tea strainer
- Coverslip
- Microscope slide.

Procedure

(1) Add 2 g of fresh feces to a container, such as a specimen container or a wax paper cup.
(2) Add flotation solution to the feces and mix well using a tongue depressor.
(3) Strain this mixture through a metal tea strainer into the second specimen container.
(4) This strained mixture is then added to the fecal shell vial (or test tube).
(5) Add more flotation solution to the shell vial until a meniscus is formed.
(6) Place a coverslip over the meniscus and let it sit for 10-15 minutes (time will vary depending upon which type of solution is used).
(7) After the allotted time, remove the coverslip by lifting it directly upwards.
(8) Place the coverslip onto a microscope slide. When laying the coverslip down, place it at an angle in order to decrease the number of air bubbles that can become trapped underneath the coverslip.
(9) Examine microscopically.

Note: It is important not to delay examination. Depending upon the type of flotation solution used, delay can result in parasite egg distortion and the solution can begin to crystallize.

There are many commercial kits available on the market that utilizes this same principle. These kits are disposable and can make clean up much easier.

Centrifugation technique

In comparison with the simple flotation method, the centrifugation technique is more efficient at recovering parasite ova from a sample. It does, however, require a little more specialized equipment.

Materials

- Two specimen containers (or wax paper cups)
- Metal tea strainer
- Tongue depressor
- Test tubes
- Flotation solution

- Coverslip
- Microscope slide.

Procedure
(1) Mix 1g of feces in 10 mL of flotation solution in a specimen container or wax paper cup until a suspension is formed.
(2) Pour the mixture through the metal tea strainer. Using the tongue depressor, press the material into the strainer to extract as much liquid as possible.
(3) Pour the liquid into a centrifuge tube and centrifuge the sample at 1500 rpm for 3 minutes (remember to always counter balance).
(4) Decant the supernatant, and add flotation solution. Mix well into the sediment. Add more flotation solution until a meniscus is formed.
(5) Place a coverslip over the meniscus.
(6) Return the tube to the centrifuge and centrifuge the sample at 1500 rpm for 5 minutes. (remember to counter balance)
   (a) *Note*: It is important that you use a centrifuge with swinging buckets, not stationary buckets. During the centrifugation process, tubes will swing out horizontally and the coverslip will be held in place (see Figure 4.4).
(7) After centrifugation, remove the coverslip by lifting straight upwards. Place the coverslip onto the slide and examine microscopically.

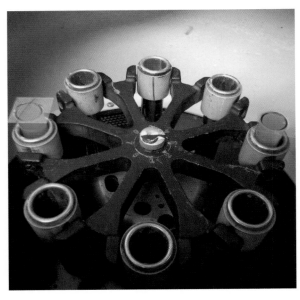

Figure 4.4 Centrifugation technique. A variable angle centrifuge is necessary for this technique.

Baermann technique

In contrast to the previous methods mentioned earlier, the Baermann Technique is used to recover parasite larvae, not ova.

Materials

- Baermann apparatus: Consisting of a funnel, support structure, short length of tubing at the end of the funnel, and a clamp at the end of the tubing.
- Gauze or cheesecloth
- Warm water
- Microscope slide
- Coverslip.

Procedure

(1) Wrap 5 g of feces in gauze or cheesecloth and lay on the support screen inside the funnel of the Baermann apparatus.
(2) After ensuring the clamp at the end of the tubing is closed, add warm water until the sample is covered.
(3) Allow the sample to sit for at least 8 hours (or overnight).
(4) After the appropriate time has lapsed, loosen the tubing clamp slightly to withdraw a large drop of liquid onto a slide.
(5) Add a coverslip to the sample and examine microscopically.

Common parasites of domestic species

Canine and feline

Nematodes

Table 4.1 *Toxocara* species: *Toxocara canis*, *Toxocara cati*, and *Toxascaris leonina* (see Figure 4.5, Figure 4.6, Figure 4.7, Figure 4.8, and Figure 4.10).

Common name	Roundworms
Host	Canine and feline
Parasite location (adult)	Small intestine
Transmission	Ingestion of parasite egg containing the larval stage of the parasite; transmission through placenta and milk
Distribution	Worldwide

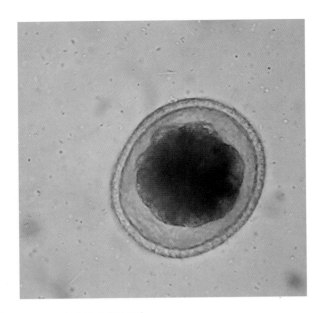

Figure 4.5   *Toxocara canis* (roundworm).

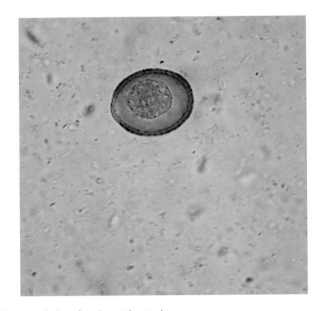

Figure 4.6   *Toxascaris leonina* (roundworm).

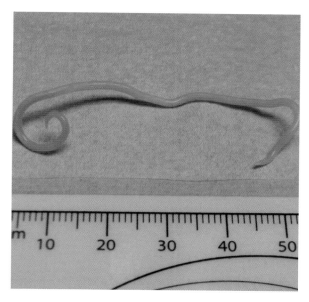

Figure 4.7 Adult roundworm.

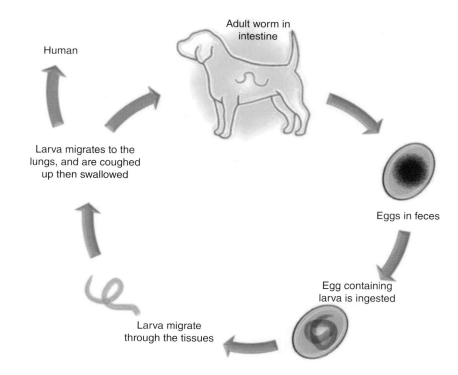

Figure 4.8 Life cycle of a canine roundworm.

Table 4.2 *Ancylostoma* species: *Ancylostoma caninum, Ancylostoma tubaeforme, Ancylostoma braziliense,* and *Uncinaria stenocephala* (see Figure 4.9 and Figure 4.10).

Common name	Canine and feline hookworm
Host	*U. stenocephala* and *A. caninum* (canine), *A. tubaeforme* (feline), *A. braziliense* (canine and feline)
Parasite location (adult)	Small intestine
Transmission	Ingestion of eggs; placental; milk; through the skin
Distribution	*Ancylostoma* spp. (worldwide); *U. stenocephala* (North America)

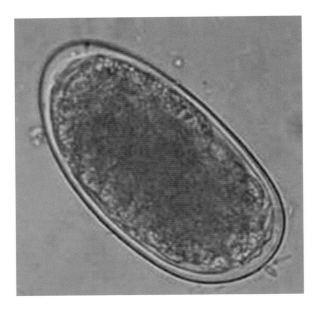

Figure 4.9 *Ancylostoma* spp.

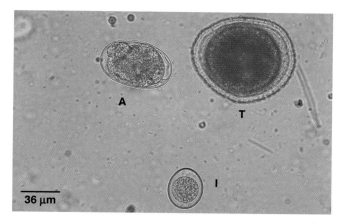

Figure 4.10 *Ancylostoma* spp. (A), *Toxocara canis* (T), and *Cystoisospora* (I) (from Zajac, Anne M. and Conboy, Gary A. 2012. *Veterinary Clinical Parasitology*, 8th ed. Ames: Blackwell Publishing).

Table 4.3 *Strongyloides* species: *Strongyloides stercoralis* and *Strongyloides trumiefaciense.*

Common name	Threadworms
Host	Canine and feline
Parasite location (adult)	Small intestine
Transmission	Milk; through the skin
Distribution	Worldwide

Table 4.4 *Trichuris* species: *Trichuris vulpis*, *Trichuris campanula*, and *Trichuris serrate* (see Figure 4.11).

Common name	Whipworm
Host	*T. campanula* and *T. serrate* (feline); *T. vulpis* (canine)
Parasite location (adult)	Colon
Transmission	Ingestion of eggs
Distribution	Worldwide

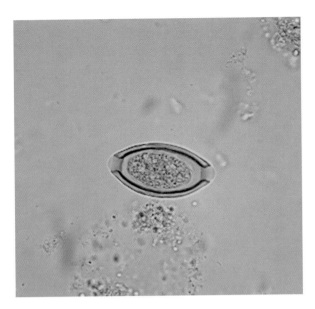

Figure 4.11 *Trichuris* spp. (whipworm).

Table 4.5 *Aelurostrongylus abstrusus*.

Common name	Feline lungworm
Host	Feline
Parasite location (adult)	Bronchioles
Transmission	Ingestion of larvae
Distribution	Worldwide

Table 4.6 *Filaroides* species: *Filaroides osleri, Filaroides hirthi,* and *Filaroides milksi.*

Common name	Canine lungworm
Host	Canine
Parasite location (adult)	Trachea; lungs; bronchioles
Transmission	Ingestion of stage 1 larvae
Distribution	North America, Europe, Japan

Cestodes

Table 4.7   *Dipylidium caninum* (see Figure 4.12 and Figure 4.13).

Common name	Double-pored tapeworm; flea tapeworm
Host	Canine and feline
Parasite location (adult)	Small intestine
Transmission	Ingestion of infected adult flea (intermediate host)
Distribution	Worldwide

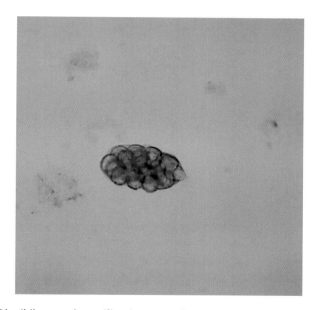

Figure 4.12   *Dipylidium caninum* (flea tapeworm).

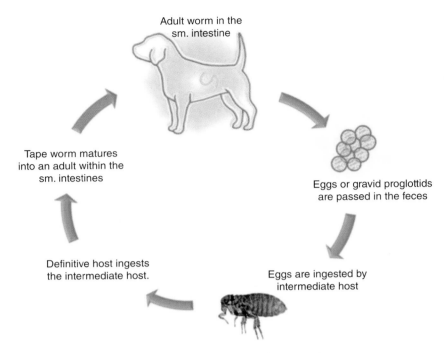

Adult worm in the
sm. intestine

Tape worm matures
into an adult within the
sm. intestines

Eggs or gravid proglottids
are passed in the feces

Definitive host ingests
the intermediate host.

Eggs are ingested by
intermediate host

Figure 4.13   Life cycle of *Dipylidium caninum* (flea tapeworm).

Table 4.8   *Taenia* species: *Taenia pisiformis, Taenia hydatigena*, and *Taenia ovis*.

Common name	Mutton tapeworm of dogs (*T. ovis*)
Host	Dogs
Parasite location (adult)	Small intestine
Transmission	Ingestion of infected intermediate host (rabbits, ruminants, and sheep, respectively)
Distribution	Worldwide

Table 4.9   *Taenia taeniaeformis* (see Figure 4.14 and Figure 4.15).

Common name	Feline tapeworm
Host	Feline
Parasite location (adult)	Small intestines
Transmission	Ingestion of infected intermediate host (rats and mice)
Distribution	Worldwide

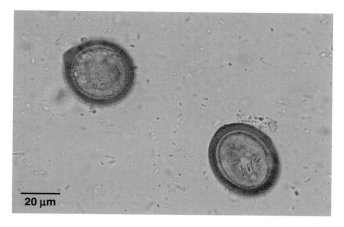

Figure 4.14 *Taenia* spp. ova (from Zajac, Anne M. and Conboy, Gary A. 2012. *Veterinary Clinical Parasitology*, 8th ed. Ames: Blackwell Publishing).

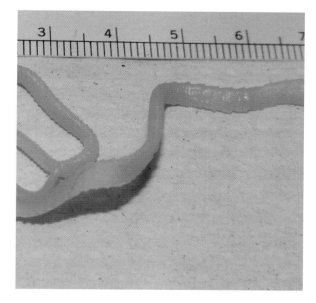

Figure 4.15 Adult tapeworm.

Table 4.10 *Echinococcus* species: *Echinococcus granulosus* and *Echinococcus multilocularis* (see Figure 4.16).

Common name	Unilocular tapeworm (*E. granulosus*) and multilocular tapeworm (*E. multilocularis*)
Host	Canine (*E. granulosus*) and feline (*E. multilocularis*)
Parasite location (adult)	Small intestine
Transmission	Ingestion of infected intermediate host (*E. granulosus*: cattle, sheep; *E. multilocularis*: rats, mice)
Distribution	Worldwide (*E. granulosus*); Northern hemisphere (*E. multilocularis*)

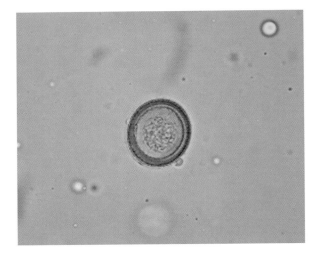

Figure 4.16 *Echinococcus* spp.

Trematodes

Table 4.11 *Alaria*.

Common name	Intestinal flukes
Host	Canine and feline
Parasite location (adult)	Small intestine
Transmission	Ingestion of infected intermediate host (frog, snake or mouse)
Distribution	Northern United States and Canada

Table 4.12 *Paragonium kellicotti* (see Figure 4.17).

Common name	Lung fluke
Host	Canine and feline
Parasite location (adult)	Lung
Transmission	Ingestion of infected intermediate host (crayfish)
Distribution	North America

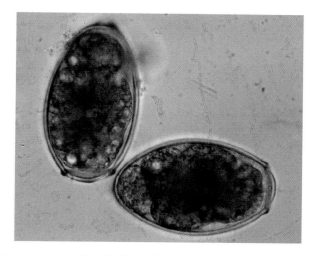

Figure 4.17 *Paragonimus kellicotti* (from Hendrix, Charles M. and Robinson, Ed. 2012. *Diagnostic Parasitology for Veterinary Technicians*, 4th ed. St. Louis: Mosby-Elsevier).

Protozoans

Table 4.13 *Giardia* (see Figure 4.18 and Figure 4.35).

Common name	Giardia
Host	Canine, feline, equine, and ruminants
Parasite location (adult)	Intestinal mucosa
Transmission	Ingestion of oocysts
Distribution	Worldwide

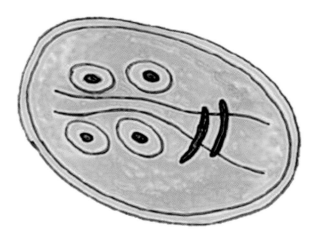

Figure 4.18   *Giardia* cyst.

Table 4.14   *Cystoisospora* (formerly *Isospora*) (see Figure 4.19 and Figure 4.10).

Common name	Coccidia
Host	Canine and feline
Parasite location (adult)	Small intestine
Transmission	Ingestion of oocysts
Distribution	Worldwide

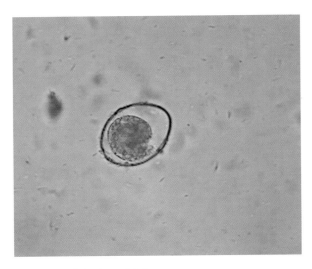

Figure 4.19   *Cystoisospora felis* (coccidia).

Table 4.15 *Toxoplasma gondii* (see Figure 4.20).

Common name	Toxoplasma
Host	Feline (can occur in other species)
Parasite location (adult)	Intestines
Transmission	Ingestion of oocysts
Distribution	Worldwide

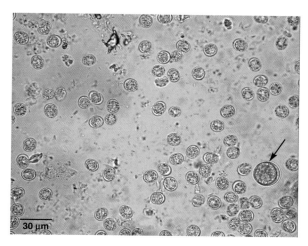

Figure 4.20 Small *Toxoplasma* oocysts. Also present is a larger *Isospora* oocyst (arrow) (from Zajac, Anne M. and Conboy, Gary A. 2012. *Veterinary Clinical Parasitology*, 8th ed. Ames: Blackwell Publishing).

Table 4.16 *Cryptosporidium* (see Figure 4.21).

Common name	Crypto
Host	Canine, feline, ovine, and swine
Parasite location (adult)	Small intestine
Transmission	Ingestion of oocysts
Distribution	Worldwide

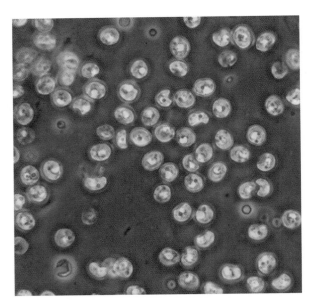

Figure 4.21 *Cryptosporidium* (from Hendrix, Charles M. and Robinson, Ed. 2012. *Diagnostic Parasitology for Veterinary Technicians*, 4th ed. St. Louis: Mosby-Elsevier).

Fleas

Table 4.17 *Ctenocephalides* species: *Ctenocephalides canis* and *Ctenocephalides felis* (see Figure 4.22 and Figure 4.23).

Common name	Flea
Host	Canine (*C. canis*); canine and feline (*C. felis*)
Parasite location (adult)	Adults found on host. Eggs, larvae, and pupae are found in the environment
Transmission	Host to host contact; contact with eggs, larvae or pupae in the environment
Distribution	Worldwide

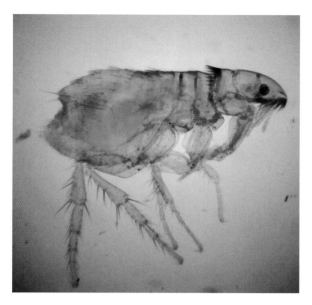

Figure 4.22 *Ctenocephalides* (flea).

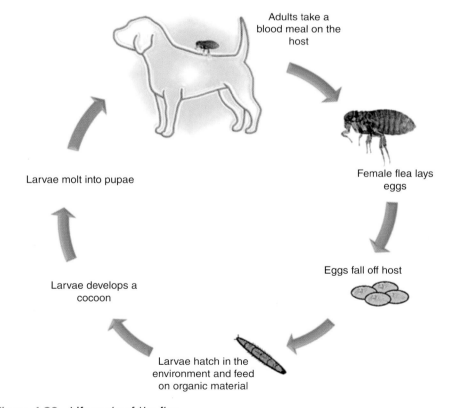

Adults take a blood meal on the host

Female flea lays eggs

Eggs fall off host

Larvae hatch in the environment and feed on organic material

Larvae develops a cocoon

Larvae molt into pupae

Figure 4.23 Life cycle of the flea.

Ticks

Table 4.18 *Rhipicephalus sanguineus* (see Figure 4.24).

Common name	Brown dog tick
Host	Canine
Parasite location (adult)	Attaches to the body
Transmission	Direct contact with infected environment
Distribution	North America
Significance	Intermediate host for *Babesia canis*

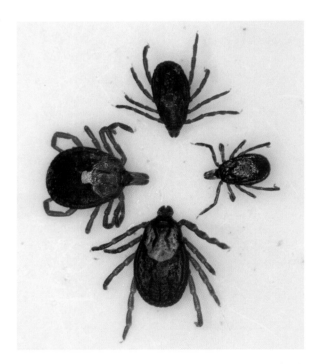

Figure 4.24 Female ticks of various species. (right) *Ixodes scapularis* (deer tick); (bottom) *Dermacentor variabilis* (American dog tick); (left) *Amblyomma americanum* (Lone Star tick); (top) *Rhipicephalus sanguineus* (brown dog tick) (photo courtesy of Dr. Susan Little, Oklahoma State University, Stillwater, OK).

Table 4.19 *Ixodes scapularis* (see Figure 4.24 and Figure 4.25).

Common name	Deer tick, black-legged tick
Host	Canine, equine, ruminants, deer, and humans (intermediate host: mice)
Parasite location (adult)	Attaches to host for feeding
Transmission	Direct contact with infected environment
Distribution	Eastern United States
Significance	Vectors for: • *Babesia microti* • *Borrelia burgdorferi* (Lyme disease) Transmits *Ehrlichia*

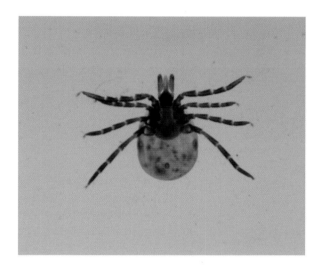

Figure 4.25 *Ixodes* spp.

Table 4.20 *Dermacentor variabilis* (see Figure 4.24 and Figure 4.26).

Common name	Wood tick, American dog tick
Host	Canine, ruminants, small mammals, and humans
Parasite location (adult)	Attaches to host when feeding
Transmission	Direct contact with infected environment
Distribution	Eastern United States
Significance	Vector of Rocky Mountain spotted fever

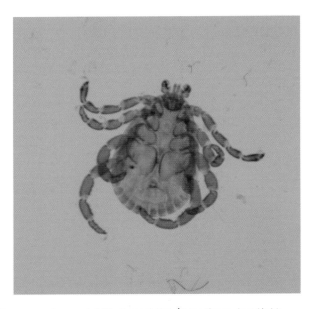

Figure 4.26 *Dermacentor variabilis* (wood tick/American dog tick).

Table 4.21 *Dermacentor andersoni* (see Figure 4.27).

Common name	Rocky Mountain wood tick
Host	Canine, equine, bovine, ovine, and humans (intermediate hosts: small rodents)
Parasite location (adult)	Attaches to the host
Transmission	Direct contact with infected environment
Distribution	Rocky Mountain regions
Significance	Vector of Rocky Mountain spotted fever

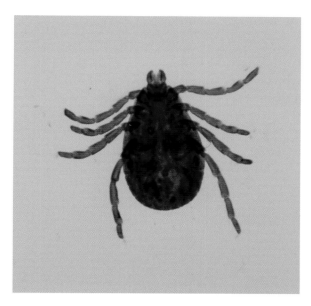

Figure 4.27 *Dermacentor andersoni* (Rocky Mountain wood tick).

Table 4.22 *Amblyomma americanum* (see Figure 4.24).

Common name	Lone Star tick
Host	Mammals, including humans (intermediate hosts: small mammals)
Parasite location (adult)	Attaches to the host. Often found near the ear
Transmission	Direct contact with infected environment
Distribution	Southern United States, Midwestern United States
Significance	Vector of: • Rocky Mountain spotted fever • Tularemia

Lice

Table 4.23   *Trichodectes canis* (see Figure 4.28).

Common name	Biting louse
Host	Canine
Parasite location (adult)	Adults, nymphs and eggs (nits) all found in the hair.
Transmission	Host to host, or via shared materials (ex: grooming tools)
Distribution	Northern hemisphere

Table 4.24   *Linognathus setosus* (see Figure 4.29).

Common name	Sucking louse
Host	Canine
Parasite location (adult)	Adults, nymphs, and eggs (nits) all found in the hair
Transmission	Host to host, or via shared materials (e.g., grooming tools)
Distribution	Northern hemisphere
Significance	Has been implicated as an intermediate host of *Dipylidium caninum*

Table 4.25 Various louse species of domesticated animals: *Trichodectes canis* (biting louse of dogs), *Linognathus setosus* (sucking louse of dogs), and *Bovicola bovis* (biting louse of cattle).

Trichodectes canis

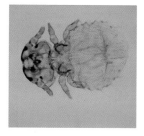

Figure 4.28   *Trichodectes canis* (biting louse of dogs).

Linognathus setosus

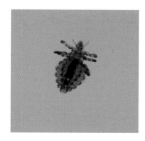

Figure 4.29   *Linognathus setosus* (sucking louse of dogs).

Bovicola bovis

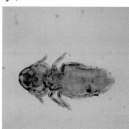

Figure 4.30   *Bovicola bovis* (biting louse of cattle).

Mites

Table 4.26   *Sarcoptes* species: *Sarcoptes scabiei var. canis* and *felis* (rare) (see Figure 4.31).

Common name	Scabies mite
Host	Canine (*canis*); feline (*felis*)
Parasite location (adult)	Mites burrow in the superficial epidermal layers of the skin
Transmission	Host to host
Distribution	Worldwide

Table 4.27   *Demodex canis* (see Figure 4.32).

Common name	Follicular mange mite
Host	Canine
Parasite location (adult)	Hair follicles; sebaceous glands
Transmission	Host to host
Distribution	Worldwide

Table 4.28   *Otodectes cynotis* (see Figure 4.33).

Common name	Ear mite
Host	Feline and canine
Parasite location (adult)	Ear canal (external)
Transmission	Host to host
Distribution	Worldwide

Table 4.29   *Cheyletiella parasitovorax* (see Figure 4.34).

Common name	Walking dandruff
Host	Canine and feline
Parasite location (adult)	Skin surface and hair coat
Transmission	Host to host
Distribution	Worldwide

Table 4.30 Various mite species of domesticated animals: *Sarcoptes scabiei* (scabies mite), *Demodex canis* (follicular mange mite), *Otodectes cynotis* (ear mite), and *Cheyletiella parsitovorax* ("walking dandruff").

Sarcoptes scabiei

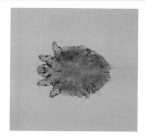

Figure 4.31 *Sarcoptes scabiei* (scabies mite).

Demodex canis

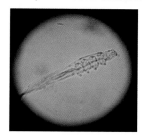

Figure 4.32 *Demoxex canis* (follicular mange mite).

Otodectes cynotis

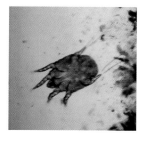

Figure 4.33 *Otodectes cynotis* (ear mite).

Cheyletiella parsitovorax

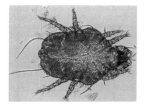

Figure 4.34 *Cheyletiella parsitovorax* (walking dandruff) (from Hendrix, Charles M. and Robinson, Ed. 2012. *Diagnostic Parasitology for Veterinary Technicians*, 4th ed. St. Louis: Mosby-Elsevier.)

Flies

Table 4.31   *Cuterebra* species.

Common name	Warbles
Host	Small mammals, occasionally canines and felines
Parasite location (larva)	Burrows into the skin. Location can be found by observing a small fistula the larva uses as a breathing hole.
Transmission	Direct contact with larva in the environment.
Distribution	North America

Ruminants

Nematodes

Table 4.32   *Nematodirus*.

Common name	Trichostrongyles with large eggs
Host	Bovine, ovine, and caprine
Parasite location (adult)	Abomasum, small and large intestine
Transmission	Ingestion of ova
Distribution	Worldwide

Table 4.33   *Strongyloides papillosus* (see Figure 4.35).

Common name	Bovine threadworm
Host	Bovine
Parasite location (adult)	Small intestine
Transmission	Ingestion of larva; penetration of skin by larva
Distribution	Worldwide

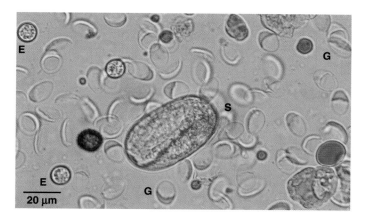

Figure 4.35   Larvated *Strongyloides* egg (S); collapsed *Giardia* cysts (G); *Eimeria* oocysts (E) (from Zajac, Anne M. and Conboy, Gary A. 2012. *Veterinary Clinical Parasitology*, 8th ed. Ames: Blackwell Publishing).

Table 4.34   *Trichuris ovis* (see Figure 4.36).

Common name	Whipworms
Host	Bovine, ovine, and caprine
Parasite location (adult)	Cecum and colon
Transmission	Ingestion of ova
Distribution	Worldwide

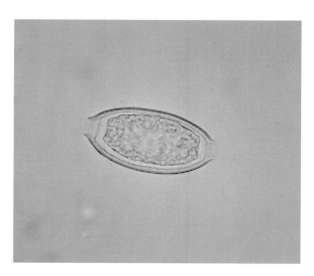

Figure 4.36   *Trichuris ovis* (sheep whipworm).

Table 4.35 *Trichostrongyle* species: *Bunostomum, Chabertia, Cooperia, Haemonchus, Oesophagostomum, Ostertagia,* and *Trichostrongylus* (see Figure 4.37).

Common name	Trichostrongyles
Host	Bovine, ovine, and caprine
Parasite location (adult)	Abomasum, small and large intestine
Transmission	Ingestion of ova
Distribution	Worldwide

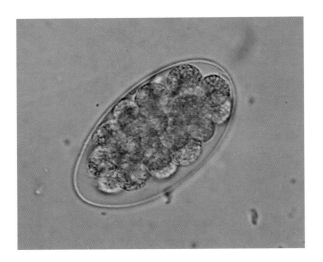

Figure 4.37 *Trichostrongyle*-type ova.

Table 4.36 *Dictyocaulus.*

Common name	Lungworm of cattle
Host	Bovine, ovine, and caprine
Parasite location (adult)	Bronchi
Transmission	Ingestion of larvae
Distribution	Worldwide

Cestodes

Table 4.37   *Moniezia benedini* (see Figure 4.38).

Common name	Ruminant tapeworm
Host	Bovine and ovine
Parasite location (adult)	Small intestine
Transmission	Ingestion of intermediate host (grain mite)
Distribution	Worldwide

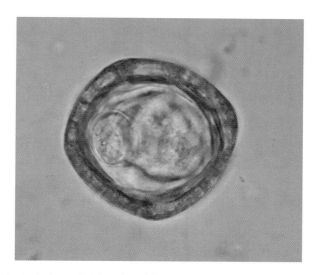

Figure 4.38   *Moniezia benedini* (ruminant tapeworm).

Table 4.38   *Thysanosoma actinoides*.

Common name	Fringed tapeworm
Host	Bovine, ovine, and caprine
Parasite location (adult)	Bile and pancreatic ducts, and small intestines
Transmission	Ingestion of intermediate host
Distribution	North and South America

Protozoans

Table 4.39 *Eimeria* (see Figure 4.35 and Figure 4.39).

Common name	Coccidia
Host	Ruminants
Parasite location (adult)	Cecum and colon
Transmission	Ingestion of oocysts
Distribution	Worldwide

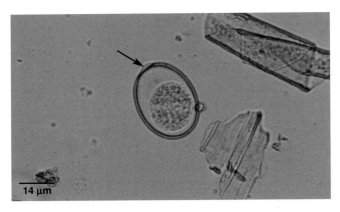

14 µm

Figure 4.39 *Eimeria* spp. (coccidia) (from Zajac, Anne M. and Conboy, Gary A. 2012. *Veterinary Clinical Parasitology*, 8th ed. Ames: Blackwell Publishing).

Table 4.40 *Cryptosporidium* (see Figure 4.21).

Common name	Crypto
Host	Canine, feline, ovine, and swine
Parasite location (adult)	Small intestine
Transmission	Ingestion of oocysts
Distribution	Worldwide

See Figure 4.21.

Ticks

Dermacentor spp. and *Ixodes* spp. have been previously discussed (see Table 4.19, Table 4.20, and Table 4.21).

Lice

See Table 4.25.

Table 4.41 *Bovicola bovis* (see Figure 4.30).

Common name	Biting louse
Host	Bovine, ovine, and caprine
Parasite location (adult)	Usually head, neck, and brisket area.
Transmission	Host to host
Distribution	Worldwide

Table 4.42 Sucking lice of ruminants: *Linognathus vituli* and *Haematopinus eurysternus*.

Common name	Sucking louse: *L. vituli* (long-nosed cattle louse), *H. eurysternus* (short-nosed cattle louse)
Host	Bovine, ovine, and caprine
Parasite location (adult)	Usually head, neck, and brisket area.
Transmission	Host to host

Mites

See Table 4.30.

Table 4.43 *Sarcoptes* species: *Sarcoptes scabiei var. bovis* and *ovis*.

Common name	Mange mite of cattle (rare) and sheep
Host	Bovine (*S. scabiei var. bovis*), ovine, and caprine (*S. scabiei var. ovis*)
Parasite location (adult)	Superficial layers of the epidermis, primarily the face in sheep.
Transmission	Host to host; fomites
Distribution	Worldwide

Table 4.44   *Psoroptes* species: *Psoroptes ovis* and *Psoroptes bovis.*

Common name	Scabies mites of sheep or cattle
Host	Ovine (*P. ovis*); bovine (*P. bovis*)
Parasite location (adult)	Skin surface; neck regions
Transmission	Host to host
Distribution	Worldwide

Table 4.45   *Chorioptes* species: *Chorioptes bovis* and *Chorioptes ovis.*

Common name	Leg mange
Host	Bovine (*bovis*); ovine (*ovis*)
Parasite location (adult)	Legs
Transmission	Host to host
Distribution	Worldwide

Flies

Table 4.46   Myiasis-producing (species in which larvae invade the tissue), biting and nonbiting flies.

Category	Scientific name	Common name
Myiasis-producing flies	*Hypoderma spp.*	Cattle grubs; heel fly
	Cochliomyia hominivorax	Screw-worm fly
	Estrus ovis	Nasal bot fly
	Lucilia, Calliphora, Phormia	Blowflies
Biting flies	*Simulium* spp.	Black flies
	Culicoides spp.	No-see-ums
	Anopheles, Aedes, Culex	Mosquitoes
	Tabanus	Horseflies
	Stomoxys calcitrans	Stable fly
	Haematobia irritans	Horn fly
	Melophagus ovinus (see Figure 4.40)	Sheep ked (wingless flies)
Nonbiting flies	*Musca domestica*	House fly
	Musca autumnalis	Face fly

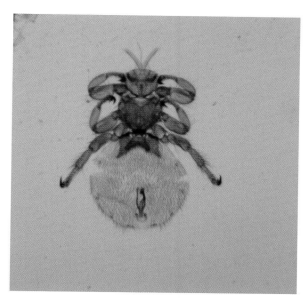

Figure 4.40 *Melophagus ovinus* (sheep ked).

Equine

Nematodes

Table 4.47 *Habronema* species (*Habronema microstoma* and *Habronema muscae*) and *Draschia* species (*Draschia megastoma*).

Common name	Stomach worms of horses
Host	Equine
Parasite location (adult)	Stomach
Transmission	Ingestion of house fly or stable fly larvae.
Distribution	Worldwide

Table 4.48 *Trichostrongylus axei.*

Common name	Stomach worms of horses
Host	Equine, bovine, ovine, and porcine
Parasite location (adult)	Stomach
Transmission	Ingestion of larvae
Distribution	Worldwide

Table 4.49   *Parascaris equorum* (see Figure 4.41 and Figure 4.42).

Common name	Horse roundworm
Host	Equine
Parasite location (adult)	Small intestine
Transmission	Ingestion of ova
Distribution	Worldwide

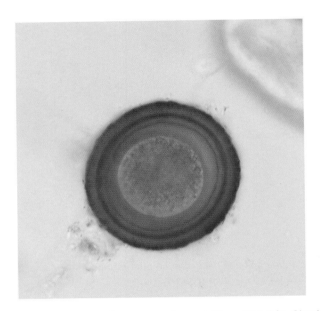

Figure 4.41   *Parascaris equorum* (horse roundworm) (from Hendrix, Charles M. and Robinson, Ed. 2012. *Diagnostic Parasitology for Veterinary Technicians*, 4th ed. St. Louis: Mosby-Elsevier).

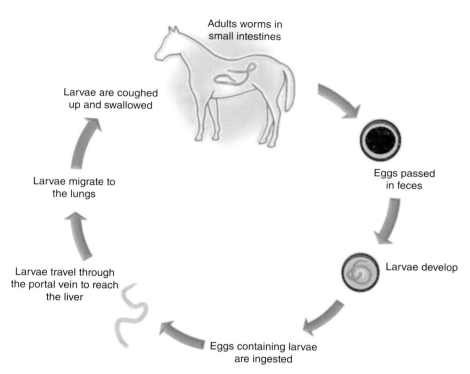

Figure 4.42   Life cycle of *Parascaris equorum* (horse roundworm).

Table 4.50   *Strongylus* species: *Strongylus vulgaris, Strongylus edentaus,* and *Strongylus equinus* (see Figure 4.43).

Common Name	Horse strongyles
Host	Equine
Parasite location (adult)	Large intestine
Transmission	Ingestion of larvae
Distribution	Worldwide

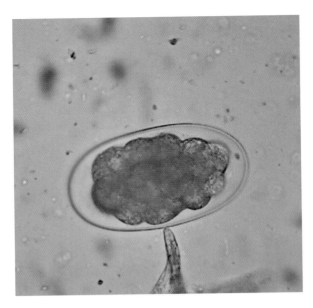

Figure 4.43 *Stongylus* spp. (horse strongyles).

Table 4.51 *Strongyloides westeri* (see Figure 4.44).

Common Name	Horse threadworm
Host	Equine
Parasite location (adult)	Small intestine
Transmission	Trans-mammary through milk; larval penetration of the skin
Distribution	Worldwide

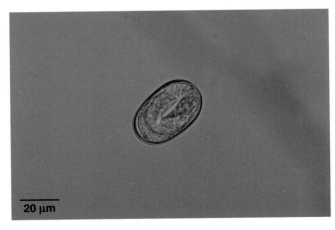

20 µm

Figure 4.44 *Stongyloides westeri* (from Zajac, Anne M. and Conboy, Gary A. 2012. Veterinary Clinical Parasitology, 8th ed. Ames: Blackwell Publishing).

Table 4.52   *Oxyuris equi* (see Figure 4.45 and Figure 4.46).

Common Name	Horse pinworm
Host	Equine
Parasite location (adult)	Cecum, colon and rectum
Transmission	Ingestion of ova
Distribution	Worldwide

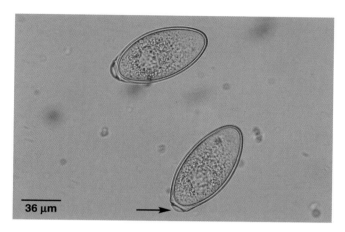

Figure 4.45   *Oxyuris* ova (from Zajac, Anne M. and Conboy, Gary A. 2012. Veterinary Clinical Parasitology, 8th ed. Ames: Blackwell Publishing).

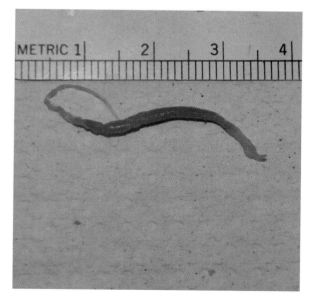

Figure 4.46   Adult *Oxyuris equi* (horse pinworm).

Table 4.53 *Dictyocaulus arnfieldi.*

Common name	Horse lungworm
Host	Equine
Parasite location (adult)	Bronchioles
Transmission	Ingestion of larvae
Distribution	Worldwide

Cestodes

Table 4.54 Equine tapeworms: *Anoplocephala perfoliata, Anoplocephala magna,* and *Paranoplocephala mamillana* (see Figure 4.47).

Common name	Equine tapeworm
Host	Equine
Parasite location (adult)	Small and large intestine (*A. perfoliata*); small intestine and stomach (*a. magna* and *P. mamillana*)
Transmission	Ingestion of grain mite
Distribution	Worldwide

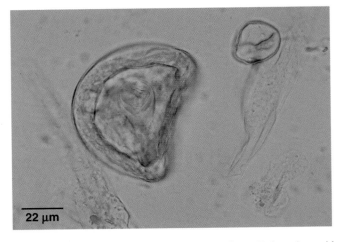

22 µm

Figure 4.47 *Anoplocephala* spp. (equine tapeworm) (from Zajac, Anne M. and Conboy, Gary A. 2012. *Veterinary Clinical Parasitology*, 8th ed. Ames: Blackwell Publishing).

Protozoans

Table 4.55   *Eimeria leuckarti.*

Common name	Equine Coccidia
Host	Equine
Parasite location (adult)	Small intestine
Transmission	Ingestion of oocysts
Distribution	Worldwide

See Figure 4.39.

Lice

Table 4.56   *Haematopinus asini.*

Common name	Horse-sucking louse
Host	Equine
Parasite location (adult)	Hair roots of mane and base of tail.
Transmission	Host to host
Distribution	Worldwide

Table 4.57   *Damalinia equi.*

Common name	Horse-biting louse
Host	Equine
Parasite location (adult)	On the body, commonly seen on the sides of the neck
Transmission	Host to host
Distribution	Worldwide

See Table 4.25.

Mites

Table 4.58   *Chorioptes equi.*

Common name	Leg mange
Host	Equine (common in heavy breeds)
Parasite location (adult)	Distal limbs
Transmission	Host to host
Distribution	Worldwide

See Table 4.30.

Flies

In addition to many of the cattle flies (see Table 4.46).

Table 4.59 *Gastrophilus* (larvae) (see Figure 4.48).

Common name	Stomach bots
Host	Equine
Parasite location (larva)	Stomach mucosa
Transmission	Ingestion of ova (attached to the hairs on a horse's leg)
Distribution	Worldwide

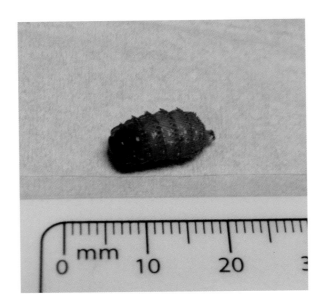

Figure 4.48 *Gastrophilus* larva (bots).

Chapter 5
Cytology

Sample collection

Swabs

Swabs are used as a collection method for sites such as body cavities or fistulous tracts. The goal of this method is to collect superficial cells or bacteria for preliminary or diagnostic cytology or culture. These cells are delicate in nature, and a gentle approach should be taken during collection. Examples of locations where this method is ideal would be the nasal cavity (i.e., looking for fungal spores) (see Figure 5.1) or vagina (i.e., establishing which phase of the estrous cycle) (see Figure 5.33).

Materials
- Cotton swabs (sterile swabs if culturing is desired or utilize a commercial culturette)
- 0.9% Saline
- Microscope slides.

Procedure

(1) Moisten the swab using 0.9% saline. Using an isotonic solution, such as saline, will preserve cell integrity and assist in microscopic evaluation.
(2) If the sample will be used for culture, a sterile swab should be used for collection and the sample stored in the appropriate culture media. When culturing an infected area, the mucopurulent secretions should be avoided, as these contain dead bacteria, yeast, microbes, and WBCs. Sampling the reddened surface of the infected tissue will yield the microbe(s) responsible for the infection.
(3) With appropriate restraint, insert the swab into the desired cavity and gently roll the swab against the mucosal surface or lining of the fistula, collecting the superficial cells. With the swab moistened, cell damage will be reduced during collection and smear preparation.
(4) To transfer the collected cells onto microscope slides, gently roll the swab along the length of the slide. Using a rolling technique versus rubbing the swab onto the slide will minimize cell damage (see Figure 5.2).
(5) Allow slide to air dry and stain.

Veterinary Technician's Handbook of Laboratory Procedures, First Edition. Brianne Bellwood and Melissa Andrasik-Catton.
© 2014 John Wiley & Sons, Inc. Published 2014 by John Wiley & Sons, Inc.

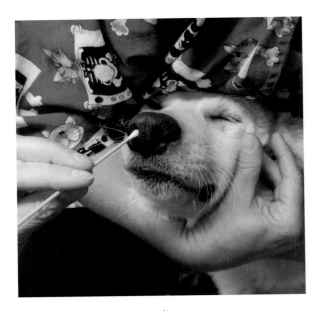

Figure 5.1   Swab collection of the nasal cavity.

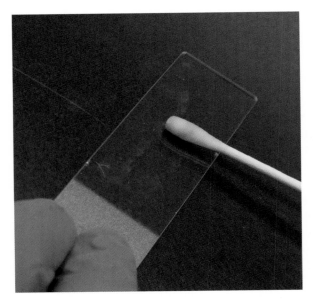

Figure 5.2   Using the rolling technique used to transfer collected material from the swab onto the slide.

Tip: Avoid using "clean stains" for this procedure, as they will become contaminated. An alternate method that will avoid this contamination is to use a pipette to flood the slide with stain versus dipping the slide into the stain itself.

Fine needle biopsy

Fine needle biopsies may be obtained from various masses, lymph nodes, organs, and nodular lesions. The principle behind a fine needle biopsy is that cells are sampled from within the target area itself, which avoids surface contaminants, such as debris, bacterial contamination, or cellular contamination.

There are two methods of fine needle biopsy collection: the aspiration technique and the nonaspiration technique.

Site preparation

The preparation required depends on the collection site and the tests to be performed. If any body cavity is to be penetrated (such as the peritoneal or thoracic cavity), a surgical prep should be performed prior to collection. If any microbiological testing is to be done, a surgical prep is also warranted. Any other sampling site requires no more preparation that that required for a vaccination or injection.

Materials
- Microscope slides
- Surgical prep materials (if required)
- 21- to 25-g needle

   Needle gauge selection is important and varies depending upon the mass. Generally, the softer the mass, the smaller-gauge needle is used. Using a larger needle often results in more bleeding. In addition to blood contamination of the sample, a large needle is less likely to collect individual cells for evaluation. Instead, it has the tendency to collect a small biopsy of tissue. For certain masses (i.e., mast cell tumors), a smaller needle, in conjunction with the added pressure of aspiration, could result in degranulation of the cells.
- 3- to 12-cc syringe

   Syringe selection also depends upon the mass. A large syringe has the potential for creating greater amounts of negative pressure. Softer masses do not require as much negative pressure as firmer masses.

   Also consider the fact that controlling the syringe during the collection procedure needs to be performed with one hand. Choose a syringe size that can be comfortably handled with one hand, yet provide you with the desired negative pressure.

Fine needle biopsy: Aspiration technique
(1) With one hand, stabilize the mass.
(2) Insert the needle into the mass.
(3) Retract the plunger of the syringe to create negative pressure (see Figure 5.3).
(4) While maintaining negative pressure and without exiting the mass, redirect the needle several times.
(5) Release the plunger of the syringe.

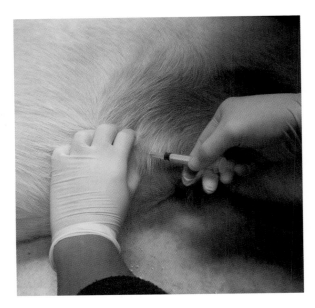

Figure 5.3 Fine needle biospy: Aspiration technique.

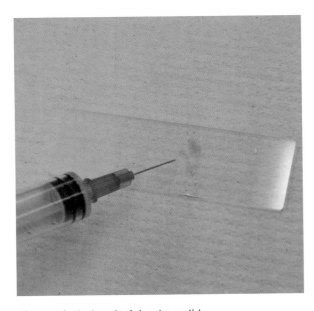

Figure 5.4 Expelling aspirated material onto a slide.

(6) Exit the mass.
(7) Remove the needle from the syringe, and fill the syringe with air.
(8) This expulsion of contents can be attempted multiple times until all cells from the needle have been expelled (see Figure 5.4).
(9) Smear the sample using desired method.
(10) Allow to air dry.

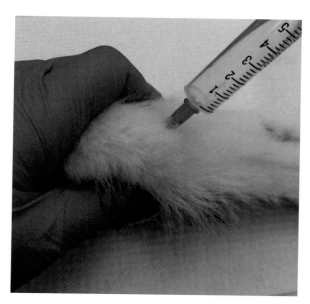

Figure 5.5 Fine needle biopsy: Nonaspiration technique.

Fine needle biopsy: Nonaspiration technique (also call capillary technique)

The Nonaspiration, or Capillary Technique is a useful method for collecting samples from masses that have a high potential for hemorrhage. One example would be gingival masses. The technique is somewhat similar, with the main difference being the lack of negative pressure used during collection. Cells are collected by capillary action and gather within the bore of the needle.

(1) With one hand, stabilize the mass.
(2) Insert the needle into the mass. Use only the attached barrel of the syringe without the plunger inserted. An alternate method is to use the needle alone (see Figure 5.5).
(3) Redirect the needle several times.
(4) Exit the mass.
(5) Remove the needle from the syringe (if using this method), and fill the syringe with air.
(6) Reattach the needle and eject the sample onto the slide as in the previous method.
(7) Smear the sample using desired method.
(8) Allow to air dry.

Tissue biopsy

A tissue biopsy involves sampling a small section of tissue, rather than individual cells. Once collected, the sample is useful for cytological or histological examination. Sites biopsied include superficial locations, such as skin or masses, internal organs (using ultrasound-guided biopsy techniques), and intestinal biopsies using an endoscope.

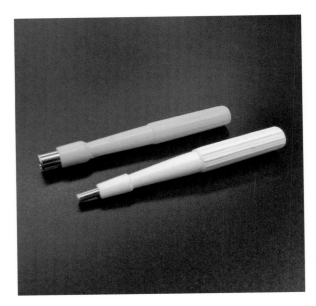

Figure 5.6   Various sizes of punch biopsies.

Site preparation

If an external mass or a skin biopsy is desired, the hair should be clipped. Cleansing or scrubbing of the site should be avoided, as it may distort elements of clinical significance.

For organ biopsies, a surgical prep is required.

Tissue biopsy: Wedge

Wedge biopsies are collected using a scalpel blade to excise a small piece of tissue. When selecting the tissue to excise, be sure the sample contains tissue from the lesion, the transition zone, and normal tissue. This will allow the pathologist to examine the microscopic features as they transition from normal to abnormal.

Tissue biopsy: Punch

A biopsy punch is a useful tool for collecting small, round biopsy specimens. Punches come in diameters from 2 to 8 mm. The punch has a circular blade that cuts easily with gentle rotation (see Figure 5.6 and Figure 5.7).

Materials

- Biopsy punch of desired size
- Thumb forceps
- Tissue scissors.

Procedure for a skin biopsy using the biopsy punch

(1) Place the biopsy punch, blade side down, onto the surface of the sampling site.
(2) Gently rotate the punch in one direction until the tissue layer has been sectioned.

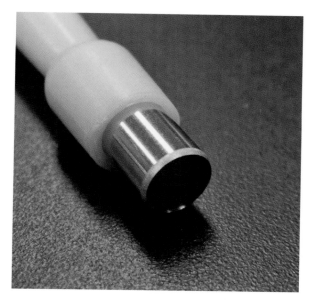

Figure 5.7   Punch biopsy circular cutting blade.

(3) Remove the punch.
(4) Grasp the edge of the sample with fine-toothed tissue forceps.
(5) Trim any subcutaneous tissue attached to the biopsy sample.

After collection, fresh imprints should be made. For histological evaluation, the sample should be fixed in 10% neutral buffered formalin.

Imprints

Imprints, or impression smears, can be made of external lesions, or of biopsies and excised masses. Superficial cells are transferred onto a slide with little cellular disruption. Keep in mind, however, that only the superficial cells are collected in this technique, and they may not be representative of the entire lesion. With certain masses, the veterinarian may have you cut the biopsy in half and make imprint slides of the inside surface as well. This will yield further cellular components that may not have been present on the superficial surface.

Procedure for external lesions

(1) For external lesions, little preparation is required. Any fluid or blood should be dabbed off prior to sampling.
(2) Place a slide face down onto the lesion and press. Do not rub or scrape the slide across the lesion.
(3) Lift the slide off and air dry before staining.
(4) Repeat this procedure a few times to create several slides for examination.

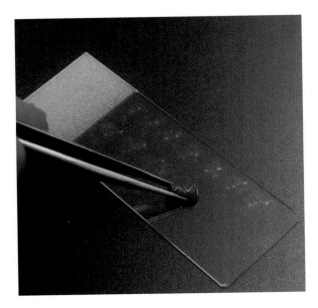

Figure 5.8 Biopsy imprints.

Procedure for biopsies
(1) A representative sample of the mass or lesion collected should be handled using forceps. Any excess blood can be gently dabbed off with gauze.
(2) Gently dab the sample several times along the length of your slide making many impressions (see Figure 5.8).
(3) If the sample is large, continue onto another slide to create more impressions.
(4) Allow slides to air dry before staining.

Centesis

Centesis is a process that involves the collection of bodily fluids with the use of a needle inserted into a body cavity. Examples include peritoneal fluid from the abdominal cavity (abdominocentesis or paracentesis), pleural fluid from the thoracic cavity (thoracocentesis), urine from the bladder (cystocentesis), joint fluid (arthrocentesis), and cerebrospinal fluid (cisternal puncture).

Site preparation
When inserting a needle into a body cavity, the site should be aseptically prepared and sterile protocols followed.

Materials
- Needle or butterfly catheter
- 6- to 60-cc syringe
- Microscope slides
- Ethylenediaminetetraacetic acid (EDTA) collection tubes and plain red top tubes.

Tip: The gauge of needle or butterfly catheter will vary with the sample collection site and the patient being sampled. A safe way to withdraw large amounts of fluid is to use an intravenous catheter. The catheter is inserted into the cavity and needle removed. A syringe is attached and fluid is drawn out.

Smears should be made immediately after fluid is collected, and any remaining fluid should be placed in EDTA and plain red top tubes. A physical examination should be made on the fluid and noting color, turbidity, and volume collected. A total protein or specific gravity should be performed on the fluid. During slide analysis, total nucleated cell counts, types, and morphological assessments should be performed.

In samples with low cellularity, a portion of the collected fluid can be centrifuged to concentrate the cellular components. After centrifugation, the sediment is examined microscopically. The remaining, unspun sample should be saved for other methods of analysis.

Scrapings

Scrapings performed on external lesions yield a high number of cells, but are limited to collecting the superficial cells only. These cells may not always be indicative of the lesion itself. They may represent normal cells, a secondary infection, or inflammation.

Materials
- No. 10 scalpel blade
- Microscope slides.

Procedure
(1) Anchor the lesion or skin with one hand for stability.
(2) Hold the scalpel blade perpendicular to the cleaned lesion (see Figure 5.9).

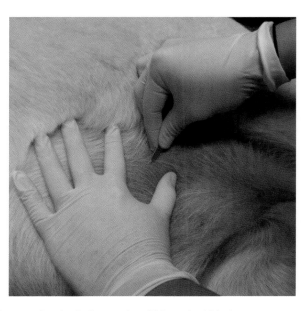

Figure 5.9 Skin scraping technique using #10 scalpel blade.

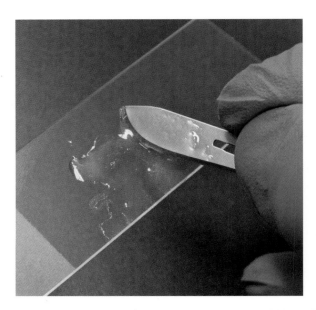

Figure 5.10 To examine the scraping for *Demodex canis*, spread the collected material onto slide and mix into the mineral oil.

(3) Scrape the blade horizontally across the tissue.
(4) Repeat this several times until a build-up of cells is seen on the edge of the blade.
(5) Spread the sample onto a slide, using the blade to thin the sample.
(6) Use the compression technique (see Figure 5.14) to make a smear.

This technique is also used in the diagnosis of skin mites, such as *Demodex canis* (see Figure 5.11). The collection procedure is the same, but when transferring the sample onto a slide, it is helpful to use a drop of mineral oil on the slide and mix the sample into it. Use the blade to thin the sample (see Figure 5.10).

Tip: To aid in the collection of cells, a drop of mineral oil can be added to the blade of the scalpel prior to scraping.

Smear preparation

Because cytological specimens vary in consistency, there are several different methods available in preparing a smear. The method should be chosen with consideration made to the thickness of the sample and the planned evaluation and staining procedure to follow. There are certain cytology collections that have a specific smear type associated with them (i.e. lymph node aspirates and various centeses would need to be smeared. Imprints from biopsies are never smeared).

Feather smear method

This method is useful in samples that are presumed to be highly cellular. The technique is the same as in preparing blood smears for hematology (see Figure 2.1). Examine the slide at the feathered edge where the cells are dispersed evenly.

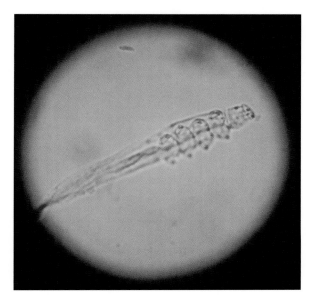

Figure 5.11 *Demodex canis*.

Line smear method

The line smear method is used in sample with a low cellular content. Cells are pushed to the end of the smear and concentrated for easier evaluation.

Procedure
(1) Add a drop of sample to the slide, near the frosted end.
(2) Using a spreader slide, back into the drop of sample and allow the sample to spread horizontally along the width of the slide (see Figure 5.12).
(3) Push the spreader slide forward, but stop before creating a feathered edge (see Figure 5.13).
(4) Lift the spreader slide up, leaving a line. This area should be examined for cellular components.

Compression (or squash) method

The compression method is used in samples that are suspected of having cellular clumps. This technique allows thicker clumps to be spread out evenly to facilitate identification. Care should be taken not to apply too much force to the slides during the process, as this could cause cell rupture.

Procedure
(1) Transfer the collected sample onto a clean slide toward the frosted end of the slide.
(2) Use a second slide, perpendicular to the first (see Figure 5.14). Lay this slide on top of the sample and allow the weight of the slide to "squash" the sample. Do not apply any downward force, as this can increase the chances of cell rupture.

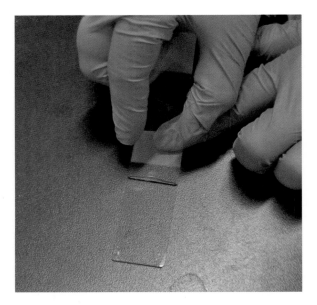

Figure 5.12   Line smear. Backing spreader slide into the drop of sample.

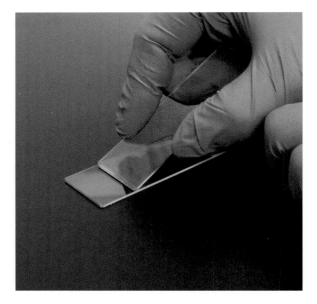

Figure 5.13   Line smear. Stopping before creating a feathered edge.

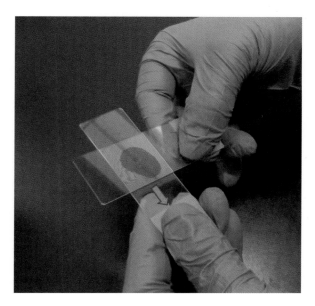

Figure 5.14   Compression smear technique.

(3) Pull the spreader slide across, smearing the sample onto its underside (see Figure 5.15).
(4) Allow the slide to air dry, then stain.

Modified squash method

The modified squash method can help to reduce the incidences of cell rupture.

Procedure
(1) Transfer the sample near the center of the slide.
(2) Add a second slide on top of the first slide, and allow the sample to squish between the two slides. As in the compression technique, do not use any additional downward force.
(3) Rotate the two slides to 45° to spread the sample (see Figure 5.16).
(4) Lift the second slide directly off of the first, and allow it to air dry before staining.

Starfish method

The starfish method can be useful to gently spread samples onto a slide.

Procedure
(1) Add the sample to the middle of a slide.
(2) Use the tip of a smaller-gauge needle to spread the material outwards in several directions. (see Figure 5.17)
(3) Allow the slide to air dry.

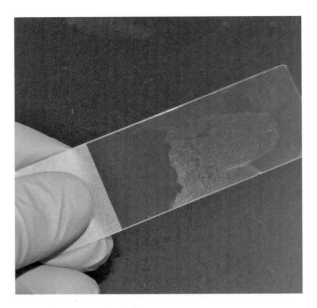

Figure 5.15 Compression smear technique.

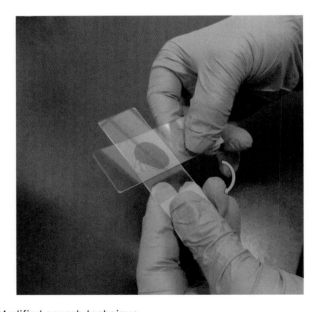

Figure 5.16 Modified squash technique.

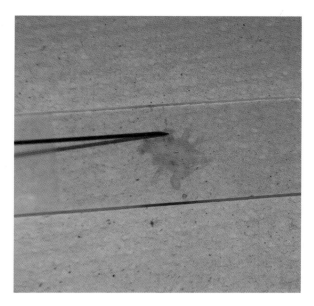

Figure 5.17   Starfish technique.

Staining

After the slide has been made, allow it to fully air dry. Avoid the use of hair dryers or open flames to speed up the drying process, as this can cause cell distortion.

The two most common staining types are Romanowsky stains and new methylene blue (NMB). Each has its own advantages and disadvantages.

Romanowsky stains (Wright's and Diff-Quick)

Romanowsky stains will stain both the cytoplasms and nuclei of cells present in the sample. While the Romanowsky stains do not provide the best nuclear detail, it is usually sufficient for the cytological determination of inflammation or neoplasia.

Regardless of the type of Romanowsky stain used, a general rule to follow is to increase the staining time when working with thicker samples.

New methylene blue

NMB stains cytoplasms weakly, but provides excellent nuclear detail. Because of this, NMB is useful in samples with high amounts of blood contamination. The red blood cells do not take up much stain and therefore will not obscure the nucleated cells when observed microscopically.

Wet mount technique (NMB)

(1) Add one drop of NMB stain to an air-dried cytology slide.
(2) Place a coverslip over the drop, and allow the stain to disperse. Let the stain sit for 2-5 minutes to facilitate stain uptake. This will result in easier examination of the cells.
(3) Examine microscopically.

Tip: **NMB stain should be filtered first to eliminate any stain precipitate that may interfere with the microscopic evaluation.**

Microscopic evaluation of cytology slides

The microscopic evaluation of a stained slide should begin with scanning under 10× objective power to locate areas where cells are evenly spaced and can easily be evaluated. Use 40× and 100× objective powers to identify, classify, and evaluate cell types.

Many familiar blood cell types will be present, and in addition, certain tissue cell types will be seen (see Figure 5.18 and 5.19).

Many cells will have undergone morphological changes associated with degeneration and disease. Pyknosis, karyolysis, and karyorrhexis should all be noted if seen.

Pyknosis and karyorrhexis

Pyknosis is associated with slow cell death (aging of a cell). Characteristics include dark, condensed, small round nuclei that may also be fragmented (karyorrhexis) (see Figure 5.20).

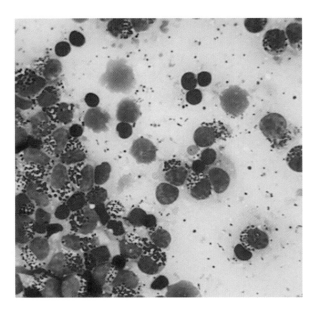

Figure 5.18   Mast cells.

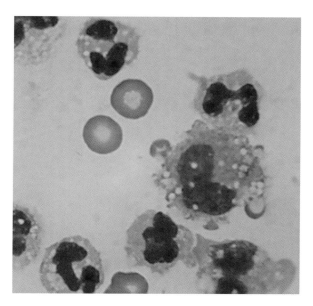

Figure 5.19   Macrophage present in peritoneal fluid (also present: degenerating neutrophils and red blood cells).

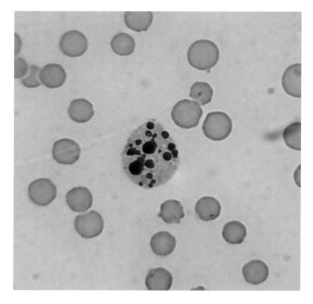

Figure 5.20   Pyknotic neutrophil displaying karyorrhexis.

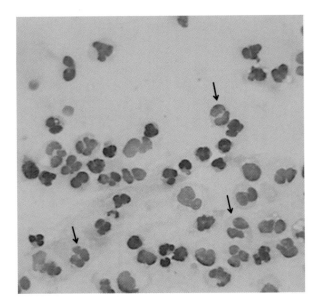

Figure 5.21   Perionteal fluid: Neutrophils displaying karyolysis.

Karyolysis

Karyolysis (see Figure 5.21) is associated with rapid cell death and is often seen in septic inflammatory reactions. Characteristics include a swollen nucleus without an intact nuclear membrane. As a result, cells portraying karyolysis have a nucleus that does not stain as intensely as other cells.

Classifying cell types

Inflammation

Cells seen in inflammatory cases include:
- Neutrophils (see Figure 5.22)
- Red cells (if hemorrhage has occurred)
- Eosinophils may be present
- Mononuclear cells, such as macrophages, lymphocytes, and plasma cells (see Figure 5.23)
- Bacteria and other microorganisms (see Figure 5.24).

The classification of the type of inflammation present can be made by the proportions of the cell types seen. Relative differential counts should be performed and cell morphology noted. Bacteria should be classified as either cocci or bacilli, and if they are single, in pairs, or chains. Comments should also be made if the bacteria were found extracellular or intracellular. Pay close attention during the slide review as certain fungal organisms can be difficult to spot.

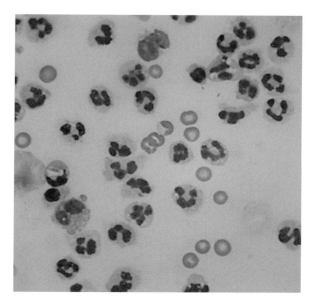

Figure 5.22   Neutrophils present in an abdominocentesis sample.

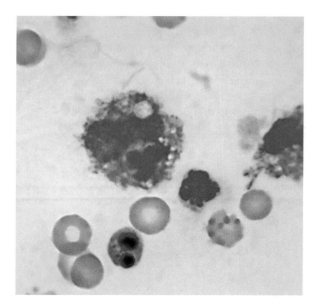

Figure 5.23   Red blood cells and a macrophage present in an abdominocentesis sample. (Note the phagocytosed neutrophil within the macrophage.)

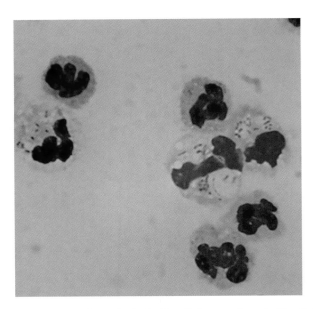

Figure 5.24   Bacteria should be noted whether it is seen free in the fluid or within the cell following phagocytosis. This is intracellular bacteria.

Other cell types

Other cell types found in cytological samples include epithelial (see Figure 5.25), mesenchymal (see Figure 5.26) and round cells (see Figure 5.27). Epithelial cells can be, cuboidal, columnar, keratinized, or squamous. They exfoliate easily and are usually seen in clumps. Mesenchymal cells are of connective tissue origin and tend to exfoliate singly. Round cells are found individually, and hold a round shape.

Neoplasia

In many cases, our cytology specimens are collected from suspected neoplastic lesions. Cells seen are evaluated for malignant characteristics. Compared with an inflammatory sample, a neoplastic sample will have a more homogenous population of cells. However, neoplasia and inflammation can occur concurrently.

Malignant characteristics
- Macrocytosis
- Anisokaryosis (see Figure 5.28)
- Pleomorphism
- High nucleus to cytoplasm ratio
- Increased mitotic activity (see Figure 5.29)
- Large or irregularly shaped nucleoli
- Coarse chromatin
- Anisonucleosis (see Figure 5.30)
- Multinucleation.

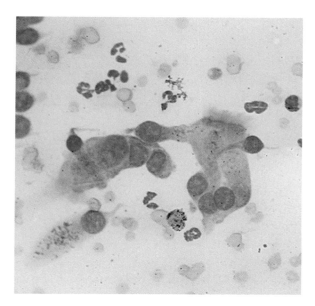

Figure 5.25   Ciliated epithelial cell (from Hendrix, Charles M. and Sirois, Margi. 2007. *Laboratory Procedures for Veterinary Technicians*, 5th ed. St. Louis: Mosby-Elsevier).

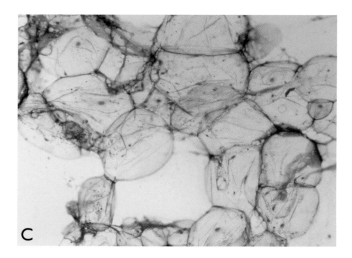

Figure 5.26   Lipoma. Mass consisting of adipocytes, which are a mesenchymal-type cell (from Rosenfeld, Andrew J. and Dial, Sharon M. 2010. *Clinical Pathology for the Veterinary Team*. Ames: Blackwell Publishing).

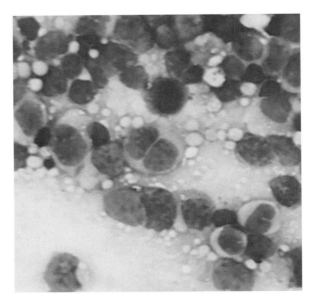

Figure 5.27   Round cells from a lymph node aspirate.

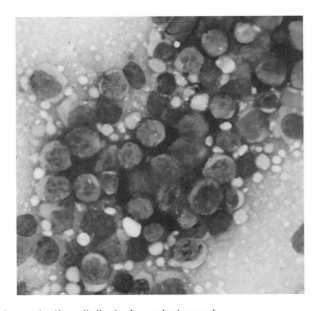

Figure 5.28   A neoplastic cell displaying anisokaryosis.

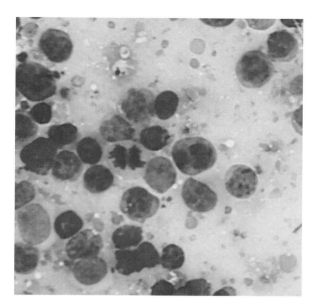

Figure 5.29   Mitotic figure.

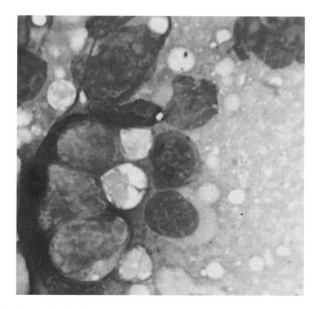

Figure 5.30   Anisonucleoliosis.

Reporting your findings

Submission of your findings should include comments on the following information:

(1) Cellularity: Low, moderate, or high (low: 0-3 cells/hpf, moderate: 3-5 cells/hpf, high: >5/hpf)
(2) Relative differential count of cell population
(3) Cellular morphology
(4) Comment on nuclear characteristics
(5) Microorganisms.

Laboratory submissions

If biopsies or slides are to be submitted to a reference laboratory for analysis, there are several important points to consider:

- Provide a detailed patient history pertaining to the lesion (duration of problem, growth rate, is the animal pruritic or painful, etc.)
- Comment on the physical appearance of the lesion. (Is it a tumor, nodule, or cyst? Is there alopecia, hyperpigmentation, etc.?)
- Describe the location of the lesion, or mark the location on a diagram. If a representative sample of a larger lesion is being sent, indicate the size of the original lesion.
- Tissue samples should be preserved in formalin prior to shipping. In northern climates, formalin may freeze during shipping in the winter months. Reference laboratories may recommend a specimen be fixed in formalin for 24 hours, and then shipped in alcohol. This procedure should be confirmed with the lab prior to shipment, and it should be indicated on the requisition form.
- Laboratories may prefer a specific type of staining for slide submissions. Slides can be submitted air dried or fixed in alcohol. This should be noted on the requisition form. If a staining procedure is used prior to shipment, this also should be indicated on the form.
- Unstained slides should not be packaged with or kept near formalin vapors. Formalin will alter the proteins within the sample, and this in turn will affect the staining procedure.
- Ensure all slides and containers are fully labeled with patient information, date, and sample type.

Ear cytology

Collecting and preparing a cytological smear of an ear sample is valuable for diagnosic purposes. Abnormal findings can include inflammatory reactions, abundance of *Malassezia* organisms, bacterial infections, or parasites like *Otodectes cynotis* (ear mite).

Slide preparation and staining

Materials
- Swabs
- Microscope slides.

Procedure
(1) Collect the samples using the swab technique, but there is no need to moisten the swab with saline.
(2) Collect the samples from the ear canal, generally where the vertical canal and the horizontal canal meet.
(3) Add the sample to your slide. Roll the sample from the right ear onto one side of the slide in the shape of an "R," and the sample from the left ear onto the other end of the slide in the shape of an "L." Using this method will aid in distinguishing differences between the left and right ear.
(4) Stain using the Diff-Quick method and examine when dry.

Heat fixing: Heat fixing is not recommended when staining ear swab slides. If there is a large amount of cerumen present on the slide, gently heating the slide by passing over a flame a couple of times can help break down the oils to facilitate staining. The gentle heating of the slide in this manner will avoid damaging cellular structures.

Modified collection procedure if mites are suspected
(1) Before collecting the sample, add a drop of mineral oil to a slide.
(2) Collect a swab sample of debris from the ear canal.
(3) Add the sample to the mineral oil and emulsify it into the oil and spread the sample so it is not thick.
(4) Examine under 10× or 40× objective for the presence of *Otodectes cynotis* (see Figure 5.31) parasites or ova.

Microscopic findings

Normal ear cytology will contain cornified squamous epithelial cells and few organisms. Abnormal findings can implicate the causative agent of the inflammation. These would include *Malessezia* or bacteria. White blood cells should not be seen on a normal or otitis externa slide. However, if WBCs are noted, this could be indicative of a middle ear infection (see Figure 5.32).

Vaginal cytology

Vaginal cytology is a useful tool in canine reproduction. Cytological changes in the estrous cycle of canines reflect the changes of estrogen throughout the heat cycle. Outward physical signs and behavior changes are also seen, but can vary among individual females. Cytological interpretation of vaginal swabs is much more reliable in determining a canine's fertile period.

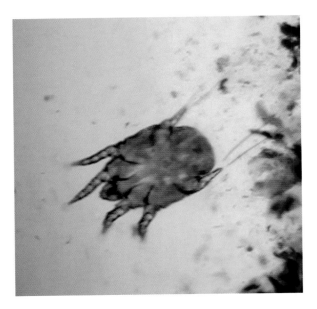

Figure 5.31   *Otodectes cynotis* (ear mite).

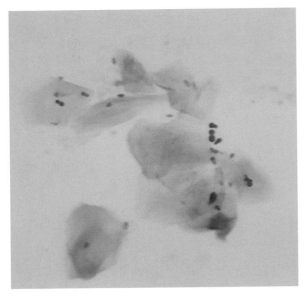

Figure 5.32   Epithelial cells and peanut-shaped *Malessezia* organisms from an ear swab.

Collection methods

Collecting vaginal samples is accomplished by using the swab collection technique.

Materials
- Swab (moistened with saline)
- Microscope slides
- Speculum (if desired).

Procedure
(1) Moistened the swab with 0.9% saline.
(2) If necessary, have someone restrain the dog.
(3) Depending upon preference, some individuals may use a speculum (or an otoscope cone) to avoid contamination with hair or debris.
(4) Insert the swab at a relatively steep angle upwards (see Figure 5.33).
(5) After the swab is inserted roughly 1 inch, lower the angle to approximately 45° and continue. Depending upon the size of the dog, the swab would be inserted anywhere from a couple of inches to several inches.
(6) Once the swab is inserted, rotate the swab two or three times then remove the swab.
(7) Transfer the sample onto the slides in the manner described in the "Swab Sample Collection" section of this chapter.
(8) Using proper slide staining techniques, stain the slide with a Diff-Quick type stain.

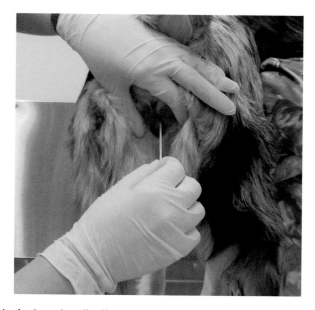

Figure 5.33 Vaginal swab collection.

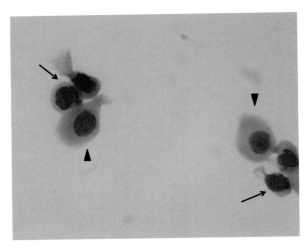

Figure 5.34 Parabasal vaginal epithelial cells (arrows) with small intermediate cells (arrow heads).

Cell types seen

The majority of the cells seen microscopically when evaluating a vaginal smear are vaginal epithelial cells. These cells are present in their various stages of development, and depending upon the stage of estrous, their proportions will vary. These cells are classified as parabasal cells, intermediate cells, and superficial cells. Other cells that may be seen are neutrophils, red blood cells, bacteria, and a few contaminating cells.

Parabasal cells
Parabasal cells (see Figure 5.34) are the smallest cells and are typically round with a high nucleus to cytoplasm ratio. They have a greater stain uptake and appear darker than the larger vaginal epithelial cells.

Intermediate cells
Intermediate cells vary in size and shape and can be further classified as small intermediate (see Figure 5.35) and large intermediate (see Figure 5.36). Small intermediate cells retain a round to oval shape with a large nucleus, while large intermediate cells begin to develop a polygonal shape with a more abundant cytoplasm.

Superficial cells
Superficial cells are the largest vaginal epithelial cells. They are thin, have sharp, angular borders and are seen with dark, condensed, pyknotic nuclei (see Figure 5.37). Superficial cells without a nucleus are referred to as cornified superficial cells (see Figure 5.38). Superficial cells may become folded or rolled up during the collection and slide preparation process.

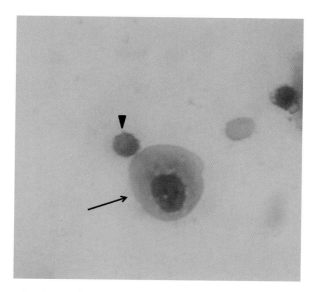

Figure 5.35   Small intermediate vaginal epithelial cell (arrow). RBCs are also present (arrowhead).

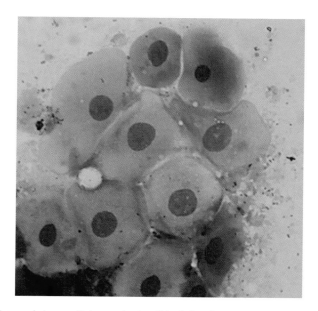

Figure 5.36   Large intermediate vaginal epithelial cells.

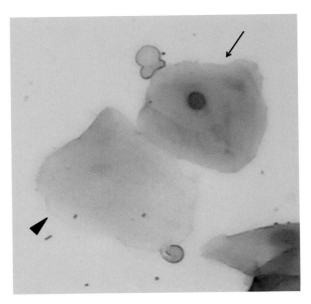

Figure 5.37   Superficial vaginal epithelial cell (arrow). Note the pyknotic nucleus. Cornified superficial cell is also present (arrow head).

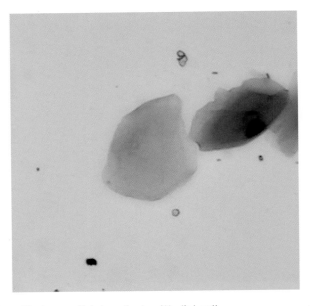

Figure 5.38   Cornified superficial vaginal epithelial cell.

Other cellular findings

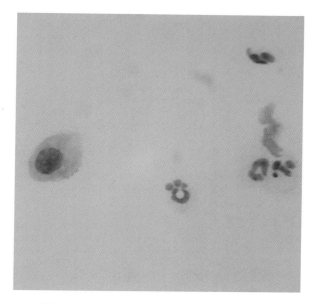

Figure 5.39   Neutrophils and a small intermediate cell present on a vaginal smear.

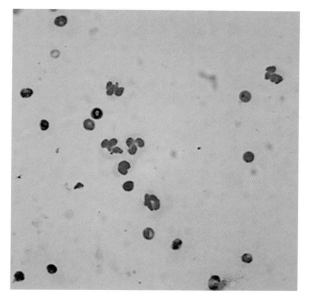

Figure 5.40   Neutrophils and red blood cells present on a vaginal smear.

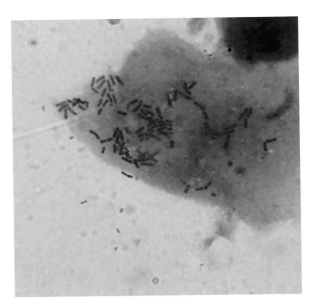

Figure 5.41 Bacteria noted on a vaginal smear. In this case, it is adhered to the surface of a cornified superficial cell.

Stages of estrous

Anestrus (duration: 3–5 months)
- Parabasal and intermediate cells predominate.
- Superficial cells are absent or present in very few numbers.
- Neutrophils may or may not be present.

Proestrus (duration: 4–13 days) (see Figure 5.42)
- In early proestrus, parabasal cell numbers begin to decrease as small and large intermediate cells predominate.
- In late proestrus, a shift from small intermediates to large intermediates and superficial cells starts to occur.
- Red blood cells are present.
- Neutrophils and bacteria are present.

Estrus (duration: 4–13 days) (see Figure 5.43)
- Superficial cells predominate, and many are fully cornified.

Diestrus (duration: 2–3 months) (see Figure 5.44)
- Dramatic decline in the number of superficial cells is seen.
- Parabasal and intermediate cells return and predominate.

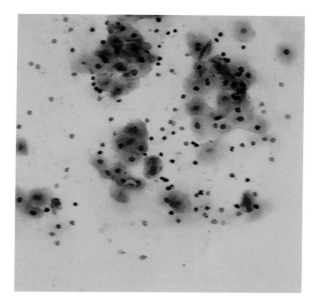

Figure 5.42 Proestrus. A mixed population of small and large intermediate cells are seen. Red blood cells are also present.

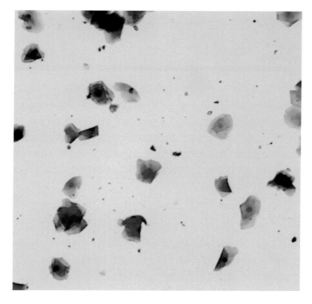

Figure 5.43 Estrus. Superficial cells make up the vast majority of the cells seen. Many are also cornified.

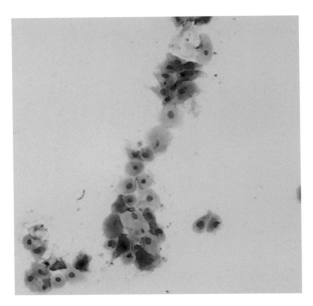

Figure 5.44   Diestrus. Parabasal and intermediate cells return. Superficial cells are absent.

Semen evaluation

Evaluating the morphology of spermatozoa in a semen sample is an important part of a comprehensive breeding soundness evaluation. After collection, the quality of a semen sample is determined based upon a number of characteristics. Volume, concentration, motility, live/dead ratio, and morphology are evaluated in conjunction with a physical and behavioral examination of the individual animal. For the purposes of this section, the focus will be on the microscopic evaluation of semen morphology and the live/dead ratio.

Slide preparation

Once the sample has been collected, a smear should be made immediately using a vital dye. An eosin/nigrosin stain is a popular vital dye for this purpose, as it provides a visual discrimination between live and dead spermatozoa.

A small drop of warm stain is added to a drop of semen on a warmed microscope slide. The two drops are mixed together and smeared. It is very important to ensure all supplies are warm. Spermatozoa are quite sensitive to cold shock, and if they are exposed to this change in temperature, a higher number of dead spermatozoa will be found. Changes in morphology will also occur. Once a smear has been made, the microscopic evaluation can be postponed to a later time. This slide can be used for both the live/dead ratio count and the morphology examination.

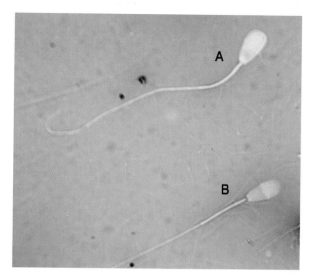

Figure 5.45   Live/dead staining using eosin/nigrosin stain. (A) Live spermatozoa appears white. (B) Dead spermatozoa absorbs the stain and appears pink/purple.

Live/dead sperm ratio

When using the eosin/nigrosin stain, determination of whether a spermatozoa is alive or dead is made by assessing the stain uptake. Live sperm resist stain uptake and appear white against the purple-stained background. On the other hand, dead sperm take up the stain and will appear pink-purple (similar to the background) (see Figure 5.45). Counts are made by examining 200 cells under 400× magnification. Live sperm counts are expressed as a percentage.

Sperm morphology

Sperm morphology can be assessed on the same eosin-/nigrosin-stained slide that was used for the live/dead ratio. The slide is examined under 400× magnification, and the morphology of the spermatozoa are evaluated, counted, and expressed as a percentage.

The anatomy of spermatozoa cell is comprised of several structures. The cell is comprised of a head, acrosome, midpiece, and tail. The tail can be further divided into the principal piece and a terminal piece (see Figure 5.46).

When evaluating morphology, any abnormalities are classified as either primary or secondary. Primary abnormalities occur during the spermatozoa cell formation (spermatogenesis). Secondary abnormalities occur at any time between storage in the epididymis to the collection and handling of the specimen. Secondary abnormalities can occur due to rough handling of the sample, cold shock or overuse of the sire animal. Primary abnormalities are considered more serious than the secondary abnormalities.

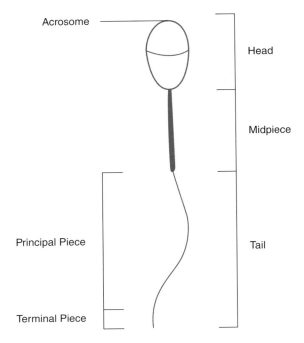

Figure 5.46   Anatomy of a sperm cell.

Acrosomal abnormalities are important to note as they are directly related to fertility. The acrosome contains the enzymes required for a sperm to penetrate an ovum. The acrosomal structure should be examined closely in frozen semen samples after the thawing process. The practice of freezing, storage, and thawing can have an effect on the integrity of the acrosome, and therefore affecting the breeding success rate (see Figure 5.49).

Primary and acrosomal spermatozoal abnormalities

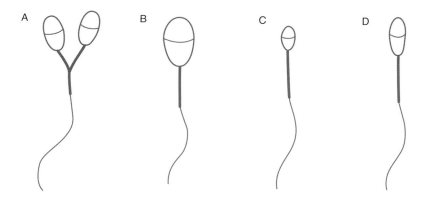

Figure 5.47 Primary cell defects: (A) double head; (B) macrocephalic; (C) microcephalic (D) narrow head.

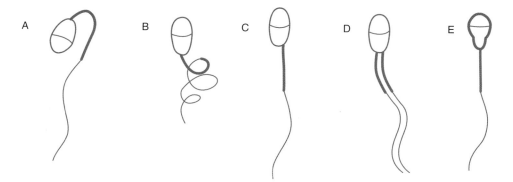

Figure 5.48 Primary cell defects: (A) bent midpiece; (B) coiled midpiece and tail; (C) offset midpiece; (D) double midpiece; (E) pear-shaped head.

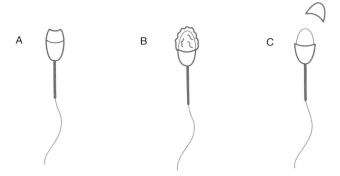

Figure 5.49 Acrosomal defects: (A) knobbed acrosome; (B) ruffled acrosome; (C) loose cap.

Secondary spermatozoal abnormalities

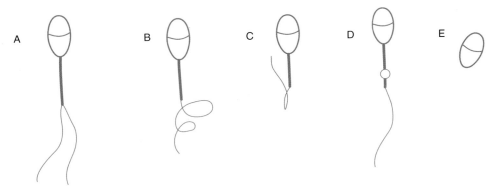

Figure 5.50 Secondary cell defects: (A) double tail; (B) coiled tail; (C) bent tail; (D) protoplasmic droplet; (E) detached head.

Appendix

Temperature conversions

$$°C = (°F - 32) \times \frac{5}{9}$$

$$°F = \frac{(°C \times 9)}{5} + 32$$

Table A.1

Degrees Celsius	Degrees Fahrenheit
36.0	96.8
36.5	97.7
37.0	98.6
37.5	99.5
38.0	100.4
38.5	101.3
39.0	102.2
39.5	103.1
40.0	104.0
40.5	104.9
41.0	105.8

Metric conversions

Length

1 m = 39.37 in
30.48 cm = 1 ft
2.54 cm = 1 in

Veterinary Technician's Handbook of Laboratory Procedures, First Edition. Brianne Bellwood and Melissa Andrasik-Catton.
© 2014 John Wiley & Sons, Inc. Published 2014 by John Wiley & Sons, Inc.

Weight

1 kg = 2.2 lbs
1 g = 0.035 oz

Volume

3.785 L = 1 gal
0.946 L = 1 quarts
29.57 mL = 1 oz
5 mL = 1 teaspoon
15 mL = 1 tablespoon

Metric system

Table A.2

Factor	Symbol	Prefix
10^{-15}	f	femto
10^{-12}	p	pico
10^{-9}	n	nano
10^{-6}	μ	micro
10^{-3}	m	milli
10^{-2}	c	centi
10^{-1}	d	deci
10	da	deka
10^{2}	h	hecto
10^{3}	k	kilo
10^{6}	M	mega
10^{9}	G	giga
10^{12}	T	tera
10^{15}	P	peta

Glossary

Activated clotting time (ACT)	A simplified version of the activated partial thromboplastin time test. Assesses the intrinsic coagulation pathway.
Activated partial thromboplastin time (APTT)	A clotting test that assess the intrinsic coagulation pathway of whole blood.
Anemia	A condition in which the oxygen carrying capacity of blood is decreased due to low hemoglobin content or low red blood cell numbers.
Anestrus	No visible signs of estrus.
Anisocytosis	Variation in red blood cell size.
Anisokaryosis	A variation of the size of a nucleus among cells.
Anisonucleosis	A variation of the size of the nucleoli within the nucleus of a cell.
Anuria	No urine formation or excretion.
Barr body	A small piece of chromatin seen during interphase of female cells. Typically seen in a drumstick shape.
Bilirubinuria	Excess bilirubin present in the urine.
Buffy coat	The middle layer of a packed cell volume that contains the leukocytes and thrombocytes.
Centrifuge	A piece of laboratory equipment designed to rotate solutions at high speeds and subjecting them to high centrifugal forces.

Veterinary Technician's Handbook of Laboratory Procedures, First Edition. Brianne Bellwood and Melissa Andrasik-Catton.
© 2014 John Wiley & Sons, Inc. Published 2014 by John Wiley & Sons, Inc.

Chromasia	Referring to the variation in cell color.
Cisternal puncture	A procedure in which a needle puncture is performed to collect cerebrospinal fluid.
Condenser	A lens system that concentrates (focuses) light into a pencil-shaped cone that passes through the specimen and enters the objective. It controls the contrast seen on the specimen
Cystitis	Inflammation of the urinary bladder.
Cytoplasm	The portion of the cell that surrounds the nucleus; may contain various organelles.
Definitive host	The host that harbors the adult or sexual stage of the parasite.
Diestrus	The period following estrus. Ovulation has occurred, and blood levels of estrogen are low and progesterone levels are high.
Diopter adjustment	Allows for the focusing of each individual ocular lens. Compensates for differences in right and left vision acuity of the user.
Dohle bodies	An accumulation of residual endoplasmic reticulum found in mature neutrophils. Associated with toxemia.
EDTA	Ethylenediamine tetraacetic acid. An anticoagulant used in blood collection tubes to prevent clotting.
Electrolytes	Inorganic compounds that disassociate in bodily fluids and carry a positive or negative.
ELISA	Enzyme-linked immunosorbent assay; used to detect or measure antigens or antibodies.
Erythropoiesis	The formation and production of erythrocytes.
Estrus	The time during the reproductive cycle when the female displays interest in mating. Ovulation is about to or has just occurred.
Fibrinogen	A plasma protein that is involved in the clotting process. Under the influence of thrombin, fibrinogen is converted into fibrin.

Frank blood	Bright red blood present on the surface of the stool.
Glomerular filtrate	The filtrate of plasma that passes through the glomerulus.
Glucosuria	Excess glucose present in the urine.
Hematuria	Presence of intact red blood cells in the urine.
Hemocytometer	An instrument used to count cells in a variety of fluids. Consist of a counting chamber etched with a grid, covered by a cover slip.
Hemoglobinuria	Presence of free hemoglobin in the urine.
Hemolyzed	Referring to the rupturing of red blood cells.
Hemoparasites	Parasites found in the blood.
Heparin	An anticoagulant used in blood collection tubes. Sodium heparin and lithium heparin are two available forms.
Hypersthenuria	Increased specific gravity of the urine.
Hypochromic	A red blood cell that has decreased hemoglobin content and therefor appear pale in color.
Hyposthenuria	Decreased specific gravity of the urine.
Icteric	A term used to describe the bright yellow coloring of mucous membranes or a plasma sample; associated with increased levels of bile pigments.
Intermediate host	The host that harbors the immature or asexual stage of the parasite.
Isosthenuria	The range of in which the urine-specific gravity equals that of the glomerular filtrate, meaning no dilution or concentration has occurred.
Karyolysis	Dissolution of a cell nucleus.
Karyorrhexis	Fragmentation of a cell nucleus.
Ketonuria	Presence of ketones in the urine.

Ketosis	Accumulation of large quantities of ketones bodies.
Kohler Illumination	Setting the microscope to align and focus the light. This maximizes both the brightness and uniformity of the specimen.
Lipemic	Referring to the presence of fatty material, or lipids, in plasma or serum.
Malassezia	A type of yeast that is often found in the infected ears of dogs and cats.
MCH	Mean corpuscular hemoglobin; refers the average hemoglobin content of a red blood cell.
MCHC	Mean corpuscular hemoglobin concentration; refers to the average hemoglobin concentration of a red blood cell.
MCV	Mean corpuscular volume; refers to the average volume of a red blood cell.
Megathrombocyte	An enlarged platelet.
Melena	Dark, tarry feces consisting of digested blood.
Meniscus	The curved upper surface of a liquid in a tube.
Microcytic	A red blood cell that has a smaller diameter than what is considered normal for that species.
Monolayer	An area of a peripheral blood smear where the blood cells are evenly distributed.
Multinucleation	A cell containing more than one nucleus.
Myoglobinuria	Presence of the muscle protein, myoglobin, in the urine.
Neoplasia	General term to describe a growth, usually a tumor; may be malignant or benign.
NMB	New methylene blue. A stain used in blood, vaginal smears, and cytology. Provides high nuclear detail.
NRBC	Nucleated red blood cell. Also referred to as a metarubricyte, these are immature, nucleated red blood cells.

Nucleus	A body within a cell that contains the chromosomes and nucleoli.
Objective lenses	The lens or series of lenses of a microscope that is nearest to the sample being examined.
Objective power	The strength or magnification of the objective lens.
Ocular power	The magnification of the oculars. Total magnification of an image is calculated by multiplying the objective magnification by the ocular magnification.
Oliguria	Decreased amounts of urine that is being produced and excreted.
Oocyst	A structure in which sporozoan zygotes develop.
Otitis externa	Inflammation of the ear.
PBS	Peripheral blood smear.
Photometry	The measurement of the intensity or brightness of light.
Plasma	The fluid portion of whole blood before coagulation.
Platelet clumping	An aggregation of platelets visualized on a blood smear.
Poikilocytosis	Referring to abnormally shaped red blood cells.
Polychromatophil	A cell displaying polychromasia.
Polychromic	A variation in the staining pattern of the red blood cell. Typically appears more purple in color.
Polyuria	The formation and excretion of increased amounts of urine.
Pooled fecal sample	One fecal sample consisting of multiple samples from multiple individuals.
Proestrus	The period preceding estrus.
Proglotids	Each segment of a tapeworm, containing a complete sexually mature reproductive system.

Proteinuria	Presence of abnormal levels of protein in the urine.
Prothrombin time (PT)	A clotting test use to measure the activity of clotting factors V, VII, and X, prothrombin, and fibrinogen.
Pyknosis	Condensed nuclear chromatin within a degenerating cell.
Pyuria	Pus in the urine.
RDW	Red cell distribution width; a measure of the variation in size of red blood cells.
Read area	The area of a peripheral blood smear where counts are performed and morphologies are assessed.
Red blood cell indices	Blood test and calculation that provide insight into the size and hemoglobin content of the average red blood cell in a sample.
Reducing agent	Substances that act as electron contributors.
Refractive index	Refers to the degree in which light will bend, relative to air, as it travels through a solution.
Refractometer	An instrument for measuring the concentration of solutes.
Regenerative	Meaning renewal. In hematology, refers to the increase production of new cells to replace the ones that have been lost.
Reticulocyte	An immature erythrocyte that no longer contains a nucleus.
Romanowsky stains	A group of eosin and methylene blue stains used in hematology and cytology. Examples include Giemsa, Wright, and Leishman stains.
RPI	Reticulocyte production index; corrects the reticulocyte count by taking into account the presence of anemia. Gives a more accurate representation of red cell regeneration.
RPM	Revolutions per minute.

Sediment	After the centrifugation process, the solution is divided into two portions. The supernatant is the liquid portion on the top; the sediment is at the bottom and consists of the solids.
Serum	The fluid portion of coagulated blood. Does not contain any coagulation proteins.
Sodium citrate	An anticoagulant used in blood collection tubes. Typically used to collect blood for coagulation studies.
Solubility	The degree of which a substance is easily dissolved.
Specific gravity	The weight of a solution as compared with distilled water.
Spermatogenesis	The formation and production of sperm cells.
Stain precipitate	Stain particles that settle out in the solution. A source of artifact.
Supernatant	After the centrifugation process, the solution is divided into two portions. The supernatant is the liquid portion on the top; the sediment is at the bottom and consists of the solids.
Trophozoites	A growing stage in the life cycle of some parasites.
Turbidity	The cloudiness of a solution.
Vacuolation	The process of forming vacuoles, or a cavity within the cytoplasm of a cell.
Volatile	Evaporates rapidly.

Bibliography

Bassert, Joanna M. and McCurnin, Dennis M. 2010. *Clinical Textbook for Veterinary Technicians*, 7th ed. St. Louis: Saunders-Elsevier.

Harvey, John W. 2001. *Atlas of Veterinary Hematology,* Philadelphia: W.B. Saunders Company.

Hendrix, Charles M. and Robinson, Ed. 2012. *Diagnostic Parasitology for Veterinary Technicians*, 4th ed. St. Louis: Mosby-Elsevier.

Hendrix, Charles M. and Sirois, Margi. 2007. *Laboratory Procedures for Veterinary Technicians*, 5th ed. St. Louis: Mosby-Elsevier.

McCurnin, Dennis M. and Bassert, Joanna M. 2006. *Clinical Textbook for Veterinary Technicians*, 6th ed. St. Louis: Saunders-Elsevier.

Osborne, Carl A. and Stevens, Jerry B. 1999. *Urinalysis: A Clinical Guide to Compassionate Patient Care*, Shawnee Mission: Bayer Corporation.

Rosenfeld, Andrew J. and Dial, Sharon M. 2010. *Clinical Pathology for the Veterinary Team*, Ames: Blackwell Publishing.

Sutton, Ted. 1998. *Introduction to Animal Reproduction: A Workbook*, Vermilion: E.I. Sutton Consulting Ltd.

Thrall, Mary Anna, Weiser, Glade, Allison, Robin W. and Campbell, Terry W. 2012 *Veterinary Hematology and Clinical Chemistry*, 2nd ed. Ames: Blackwell Publishing.

Zajac, Anne M. and Conboy, Gary A. 2012. *Veterinary Clinical Parasitology*, 8th ed. Ames: Blackwell Publishing.

Veterinary Technician's Handbook of Laboratory Procedures, First Edition. Brianne Bellwood and Melissa Andrasik-Catton.
© 2014 John Wiley & Sons, Inc. Published 2014 by John Wiley & Sons, Inc.

Index

Note: Italicized page locators indicate figures/photos; tables are noted with t.

Veterinary Technician's Handbook of Laboratory Procedures, First Edition. Brianne Bellwood and
Melissa Andrasik-Catton.
© 2014 John Wiley & Sons, Inc. Published 2014 by John Wiley & Sons, Inc.

Keep up with critical fields

Would you like to receive up-to-date information on our books, journals and databases in the areas that interest you, direct to your mailbox?

Join the **Wiley e-mail service** - a convenient way to receive updates and exclusive discount offers on products from us.

Simply visit **www.wiley.com/email** and register online

We won't bombard you with emails and we'll only email you with information that's relevant to you. We will ALWAYS respect your e-mail privacy and NEVER sell, rent, or exchange your e-mail address to any outside company. Full details on our privacy policy can be found online.

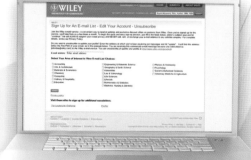

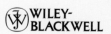
WILEY-BLACKWELL

www.wiley.com/email

17841